Citizens, Consumers and the NHS

Capturing Voices

Christine Hogg

palgrave
macmillan

First published 2009 by
PALGRAVE MACMILLAN

Palgrave Macmillan in the UK is an imprint of Macmillan Publishers Limited, registered in England, company number 785998, of Houndmills, Basingstoke, Hampshire RG21 6XS.

Palgrave Macmillan in the US is a division of St Martin's Press LLC, 175 Fifth Avenue, New York, NY 10010.

Palgrave Macmillan is the global academic imprint of the above companies and has companies and representatives throughout the world.

Palgrave® and Macmillan® are registered trademarks in the United States, the United Kingdom, Europe and other countries.

ISBN-13: 978–0–230–5063–6
ISBN-10: 0–230–55063–0

This book is printed on paper suitable for recycling and made from fully managed and sustained forest sources. Logging, pulping and manufacturing processes are expected to conform to the environmental regulations of the country of origin.

A catalogue record for this book is available from the British Library.

10 9 8 7 6 5 4 3 2 1
18 17 16 15 14 13 12 11 10 09

Printed and bound in China

This book is dedicated to the usual suspects

Contents

List of Boxes

Acknowledgements

The Economic and Social Research Council (Grant Number RES-000-22-1654) funded the research for this book and I am very grateful for the opportunities this support gave me. I am also grateful to the London Metropolitan University for facilitating this, in particular Ian Waller and Bill Bowring, Human Rights and Social Justice Institute. Special thanks must go again to Eileen O'Keefe whose enthusiasm encouraged me to undertake this research and write this book.

Foremost I want to thank the people who I interviewed as part of the research. They were generous with their time and in sharing experiences about events, which often had been personally difficult and distressing.

I would also like to thank Mike Gerrard who generously shared his own research on community health councils. I owe thanks to many other people, and would in particular like to thank Malcolm Alexander, Judith Allsop, Rob Baggott, Sally Brearley, Andrew Craig, Beryl Furr, Frances D'Souza, David Gilbert, Sally Hogg, Eileen Lepine, Anne Murcot, Naomi Pfeffer, Belinda Pratten, Jill Procter, Barrie Taylor, Charlotte Williamson and Fedelma Winkler. And of course Lynda Thompson and Sarah Lodge at Palgrave Macmillan.

List of Abbreviations

ACHCEW	Association of Community Health Councils for England Wales
AHA	Area health authority
CHC	Community health council
CPPIH	Commission for Patient and Public Involvement in Health
DHA	district health authorities
DHSS	Department of Health and Social Security
DMT	District management team
FPC	Family practitioner committee
FSO	Forum support organisation
HAS	Health Advisory Services
ICAS	Independent complaints advocacy service
LHC	Local health council (Scotland)
MIND	National Association for Mental Health
MENCAP	National Association for people with learning disability and their families
MSP	Member of the Scottish Parliament
NICE	National Institute for Health and Clinical Excellence
NHS	National Health Service
NPSA	National Patient Safety Agency
LINks	Local involvement networks
OSC	Overview and scrutiny committee
PALS	Patient advice and liaison service
PCT	Primary care trust
PFI	Private Finance Initiative
PPI	Patient and public involvement
RAWP	Resource Allocation Working Party
RHA	Regional health authority
SHC	Scottish Health Council
TAB	Transition Advisory Board

Personal Note

For most of the period covered by this book I was actively involved in many of the events described. It would be disingenuous to claim that this book is purely an academic treatise on the development of national policies on user involvement over the last 30 years. Readers may find the book shifts between an academic analysis and a personal view of the events. I hope this enhances rather than hinders an understanding of the story that it tells and the lessons that can be learnt.

I was the Community Health Council (CHC) Secretary in Kensington, Chelsea and Westminster South District from 1974–1980. From 1984 as a self-employed consultant, I worked for individual CHCs, Association of Community Health Councils for England Wales (ACHCEW) and the Society of CHC Staff, including facilitating reviews, producing training materials, good practice guides and, in the 1990s, performance standards and review of staffing levels. I also have worked for patient and consumer organisations on user involvements, charters, regulation and complaints.

During the period of transition and the abolition of CHCs, I was commissioned to look at what arrangements might be needed at national level with the abolition of ACHCEW and later became project manager for the Transition Advisory Board. Following that I worked with the Commission for Patient and Public Involvement in Health to develop guidance for forums. In 2004 I was commissioned by the Department of Health and the Commission for Patient and Public Involvement in Health to consult stakeholders about new arrangements that might be developed to replace Commission for Patient and Public Involvement in Health (CPPIH) when its abolition was announced.

Christine Hogg

The Research

This book is based on research undertaken as part of a study funded by the British Economic and Social Research Council Grant Number RES-000-22-1654. The aims of the research were to provide insights into the development of patient and public involvement in national policy 1974–2004 in the context of changing government policies. The objectives were to:

- Document the transitional arrangements leading up to the abolition of CHCs and its national body, the Association of CHCs of England and Wales (ACHCEW) and setting up of the Commission for Patient and Public Involvement in Health.
- Identify the key debates around the arrangements for patient and public involvement in national and local policy-making.
- Analyse these findings within the framework of theories of civil renewal and active citizenship, public participation and community engagement.

Documents at national level were analysed, in particular on community health councils and the work of ACHCEW, including files and documents from the archives of the ACHCEW. Information was obtained under the Freedom of Information Act from the Department of Health and the Commission for Patient and Public Involvement in Health. Archives from CHCs are available at the Wellcome Library, Oxford Brookes University and the London Metropolitan Library.

Twenty five face-to-face interviews and six phone interviews were undertaken with key people involved in the transition and implementation of policy from 2000 in order to corroborate the events outlined in the documentation and gain an understanding of the different perceptions of these events. Notes were made of each interview and these were agreed with the informant. Some informants provided sensitive information that was not recorded. It had been expected that there would be very different versions of events from people involved from different perspectives. In general this was not the case. There was agreement about events and facts, though the interpretations differed and informants had a partial views of events. The events were complex and emotionally charged and many informants found the sequence of events difficult to recall. Where there were gaps, attempts were made to clarify with other people, who were not formally interviewed as part of the research. Additional phone interviews were undertaken to clarify specific areas and check accounts provided. At the same time there were major changes in national polices in Scotland and Northern Ireland and the research was extended to include this.

Department of Health – civil servants (4), ministers (2); Commissioner for Patient and Public Involvement in Health – Commissioners (4), senior management (1), regional managers (2); Association for CHCs for England and

Wales: Directors (4), Chair (1), Management Committee (3), regional associations (1); Other agencies (2) Healthcare Commission, NHS Confederation; Northern Ireland (2), Wales (2) Scotland (5).

Introduction

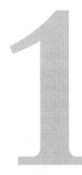

> '*The ambiguity attached to participation has helped to foster its own cause. Because so many different hopes have been linked with it, so many different expectations about what it will achieve, it has been embraced by spokesmen of highly varying political hues. Consumers have advocated participation in order to achieve their particular ends and the service providers have similarly welcomed it in order to serve theirs. The very uncertainty of its impact has enabled a common rallying call*'. Ann Richardson, 1983: 99.

Patient and public involvement has become a rallying call in the political arena, seen as part of the solution to the problems facing health services in the industrialised world. The demand for and costs of medical treatments are increasing. People are living longer, but often with chronic conditions. The expectations of affluent people are greater and they expect public services to be designed to meet their individual needs. All Western health systems are realising that there are not the economic resources to meet these demands indefinitely. Meanwhile inequalities both within and between countries are increasing.

The need to take account of the views of users and citizens is a consistent theme of healthcare reform throughout wealthy developed countries, but there is limited insight or evidence about how people should be involved or how it actually improves health outcomes (WHO, 2006). While everyone agrees that involving lay people in healthcare decisions is 'good', there are different underlying philosophies about the relationship of citizens to the state (see Box 1.1). The enthusiasm for user involvement is based on political views rather than evidence of impact (Box 1.2).

There is more support for the theory of user involvement than for its implementation. Over the last 30 years different approaches to participation have been pursued and dropped as the perceived needs of governments and the National Health Service (NHS) have changed. Policy changes are outlined in the chronology at the end of the chapter. Throughout there has been a persistent confusion about whether government wants to involve people in order to provide better health services or to involve them as citizens as part of the democratic process. Is it in order to promote democratic accountability? To

---

Box 1.1   What is in a name?

The words we choose to use to describe the lay person – citizen, customer, consumer, patient, service user or client represents a particular viewpoint and has good and bad connotations.

People themselves when receiving healthcare tend to see themselves as patients, but the term can be seen as demeaning, implying a passive role.

The term '**consumer**' or '**customer**' focuses on the individual as a more active player but no one sees themselves as consumers or customers, and it does not accurately reflect the experience of receiving healthcare, which is not just another product or service in the market.

Most people do not see themselves as '**users**' and the term can be confused with problem drug and alcohol users.

Some people who have experienced mental health services prefer to describe themselves as '**survivors**' of the system.

In looking at collective involvement there are also different terms. '**Lay**' people are defined in relation to professionals and the expertise that they do not have. The term '**citizen**' implies rights, which the more diffuse word '**public**' does not, but excludes migrants.

Bearing in mind these difficulties, the terms used in this book may vary with the context.

Box 1.2   Evidence for effectiveness

There is an extraordinary dearth of evidence about the outcomes of involvement and commentators rely on the writer's view of what worked and what did not.

In 2002 a systematic review identified 337 studies about involving patients in planning and developing healthcare, but only 12 percent described the effects and changes resulting from involvement and none examined the impact these changes might have had for other users. None used comparative or experimental research methods. The evidence that there was, supported the view that patients had contributed to changes across a wide range of different settings. Perhaps the greatest impact of user involvement is in a change of culture, which is hard to measure.

Source: Crawford et al., 2002.

---

challenge social inequalities? To promote active citizenship? To improve patients' experiences? To promote the market through consumerism and choice? To encourage self-reliance and personal responsibility? To legitimate decisions about priorities and rationing of treatment and healthcare? This confusion may have contributed to the failure of policies to involve patients and the public and limited the influence that people, as patients and citizens have on the development of health and social care.

This book explores changing policies on user involvement over the last 30 years in the UK. It examines the life and death of community health councils (CHCs) and subsequent attempts to put structures in place to enable user voices in health and social care.

Origins in social rights

Many different concerns came together in the 1960s and early 1970s to lead governments to believe that increased lay involvement, in the form of community health councils, might help solve many of the problems facing the NHS. Governments were frustrated by the failure of the NHS to implement national policies at local level and address inequalities in the distribution of resources between geographical areas or between acute and long-term care. More local involvement might help reduce these inequalities, address the democratic deficit in the NHS, increase the involvement of volunteers in the NHS and improve the co-ordination of services and planning between the NHS and local authorities.

Improving access and reaching all parts of the community was one of the expectations of community health councils when they were established in 1974. It was recognised that those most in need were not benefiting from the new welfare state. The NHS was based on every citizen having social rights, and citizens were entitled to benefits, such as free healthcare, which were not charity. Among the many expectations of CHCs, it was hoped that they would strengthen the voices of the public in the NHS, particularly those who were seen as benefiting least from their social rights. Early verdicts were that CHCs were a qualified success but needed strengthening. CHCs continued until 2003 but were increasingly struggling with the changes in the NHS and limited resources (Chapters 2, 3 and 4).

Another objective of introducing more lay involvement in 1974 was to achieve greater accountability and address the democratic deficit in the NHS. In the 1980s and 1990s CHCs lost their monopoly and many different consultation methods were used by the NHS and local authorities. In 2001 all NHS bodies were given a duty to consult and local government given powers of scrutiny of the NHS. Overview and scrutiny committees were set up, taking over some of the functions of CHCs. However, it was increasingly clear that there were more fundamental problems in representative democracy that these approaches did not address (Chapter 5).

The rise of consumer rights

The world changed with the development of management approaches in the 1980s and the market in the 1990s and governments wanted different things from user involvement. In 1979 the Labour Government of James Callaghan was replaced by a Conservative Government. The new Prime Minister, Margaret Thatcher, had very different ideas about how to tackle the problems of the NHS and the relationship of citizens to the state. Social rights on which the welfare state was based were questioned. The New Right considered that promoting social rights had undermined good citizenship by weakening personal responsibility.

With the introduction of general management in the 1980s and the internal market in the 1990s, governments saw the possibilities of using individual consumers as levers for change. It was assumed that the consumer can make choices and help to promote the market and improve the efficiency of public services. Complaints and legal action became a way of expressing dissatisfaction about the quality of services but also to get the services consumers wanted. Consumerist rather than democratic approaches became important. Consumerism, however, can undermine citizenship and increase inequalities. There was a move away from social rights to give individuals a bigger role in looking after their own health (Chapter 6).

This retreat from universal benefits and social rights was also reflected in public health policies. There has long been a struggle between those who want the state to intervene to protect citizens by reducing environmental, social and economic factors that damage people's health and lead to inequalities; and those who feel that it is up to the individual to make their own lifestyle choices. In the 1980s the government also encouraged individuals taking responsibility for their own health. This permeated all social policies and affected eligibility to benefits, including health and social care. The values of Thatcher's government resurrected the concept of the 'deserving' and 'undeserving poor'. Citizens could no longer expect social rights. They were to be earned.

Increasingly NHS policies focus on the individual and what help they need to make healthy choices, rather than the actions that government can take to make these choices easier. Holding people responsible for their own health, like consumerism, is likely to increase inequalities in health between individuals and communities. Approaches that work with communities are more likely to increase participation and engagement to those who suffer the poorest health in society (Chapter 7).

Reform and New Labour

The Labour Government came to power in 1997. In July 2000 the *NHS Plan* was published. This was a comprehensive plan promising financial investment and modernisation (DH, 2000). The most controversial policies were those relating to patient and public involvement, in particular the abolition of CHCs.

However, CHCs still had support at national and local levels and the process of abolishing CHCs was tortuous, acrimonious and distressing. During the passage of the Health and Social Care Act through Parliament, CHCs fought a successful battle and the clauses relating to the abolition of CHCs were removed. However, the framework was in place to transfer the functions of CHCs to new bodies: overview and scrutiny committees, independent complaints advocacy (ICAS) and patient advice and liaison services. All NHS bodies were given a duty to consult. The NHS and Healthcare Professions

Act that was passed in May 2002, abolished CHCs and set up patients' forums and Commission for Patient and Public Involvement in Health as a non-departmental public body (Chapter 8).

After the abolition of CHCs in 2003, patient and public involvement in England became complex and fragmented. There was a desire to recruit new people not previously involved and get away from people who were pejoratively referred to as the 'usual suspects' – that is people who were already involved in CHCs or voluntary organisations. However, forums were based on institutions and with few members, with little guidance and support, they failed. In July 2004 as part of the review of arms length bodies it was announced that CPPIH would be abolished. The abolition of patients' forums was announced in 2006. There were many reasons for the failure of the new Commission, but underlying them was a confusion of consumerist and democratic approaches to user involvement. Meanwhile CHCs remained in Wales and were reformed while in Scotland and Northern Ireland different models for patient and public involvement were introduced (Chapter 9).

Engaging citizens and social rights

Thinking within the Government had moved on even before patients' forums were established. Increasingly it was recognised that the problems of citizen engagement were broader than just the democratic deficit in the NHS and lay with representative government itself. Decision-making was devolved downward within a national framework. There was a search for new forms of democratic participation, including foundation trusts, petitions and e-democracy. Local involvement networks (LINks) replaced patient and public involvement forums, basing patient and public involvement in the context of neighbourhoods, rather than institutions and provide opportunities to integrate participation in health and social care with wider citizen engagement (Chapter 10).

Perhaps the major failure in policy has been the failure to understand the context in which decisions are made by individuals and communities in relation to their health. Many factors influence our health – individual factors such as our age, sex and genes, how we live, our social and community networks and the general socio-economic, cultural and environmental conditions of our lives. In reality the control we have as individuals over factors that affect our health is limited. Arrangements to involve people do not take these wider determinants of health into account. They address lifestyles and personal factors and target healthcare services, but do not address the big questions of both health improvement for the whole population and equity. These need to be supported by action from employment, housing, agriculture and living and working conditions.

Participation can increase inequalities. If user involvement is to promote public health, all people need to be involved and their voices heard. Formal arrangements for involvement can exclude those who do not speak out or who are not part of established networks. Involving those who are not normally involved has proved elusive. There are reasons why they are 'hard to reach'. Involving them requires addressing the inequalities, that is the health-damaging differences that people face in their lives. It also involves tackling the inequities in society, that is the injustice involved in these inequalities.

Although these different approaches have provided more opportunities for participation, there are questions as to whether they will either promote the health of the nation or improve health and social care. There has been an increasing trend towards the management of the processes of participation, Voices and views are invited on the terms of the commissioners and providers of services. Participation emerges as a process to be 'captured', managed and controlled, as part of the consumer agenda, rather than the democratic one. There is also a catch 22: those who put themselves forward as volunteers can soon be criticised as 'the usual suspects', while, those who do not volunteer, can be accused of apathy.

Participation, and this book argues, needs to be put in the context of tackling inequalities and prompting equity; ensuring access for all, based in social rights and community development approaches. A framework for social rights enshrined in law is needed for public services to engage with communities effectively, especially those that are marginalised (Chapter 11).

User involvement in health – chronology of events

Year	Events
1969	Report of the Commission of Inquiry into Ely Hospital, Cardiff identified serious neglect and abuse of patients in a long stay hospital for people with learning disabilities where professionals and the lay managers had failed to protect them.
973	NHS Reorganisation Act 1973 introduced and new administrative structure and established community health councils.
1976	**Oil crises halt expansion of public services and public expenditure of post-war years.**
	Resource Allocation Working Party Report (RAWP) aimed to allocate recourse according to health need and population.
	Prevention and Health Everybody's Business was the first public health strategy.
1979	**Conservative Party elected with Margaret Thatcher as Prime Minister.**
	Royal Commission on the NHS proposed the administrative reform and the strengthening of CHCs.
	Patients First – Consultative Paper proposed administrative reorganisations and questioned the continued need for CHCs.
1980	Black Report on Health Inequalities provided evidence of the impact of social inequalities on health.
1983	Griffiths Report, NHS Management Inquiry introduced general management and business models for public services.
1988	**Commission into citizenship set up following concerns about alienation and antisocial behaviour.**
1989	*Working for Patients* – White Paper proposed separating the functions of purchasing and providing with self governing trusts and fundholding GPs.
1990	NHS and Community Care Act 1990 separated the function of purchasing and providing services and set up framework for the internal market.
1991	Patients Charter outlined individuals' rights and standards they should expect.

User involvement in health – chronology of events – *continued*

Year	Events
1992	*Local Voices* encouraged health authorities to engage in a dialogue with community and voluntary groups.
	Health of the Nation – health strategy highlighting the impact of non-health sectors on health status and set public health targets.
	Regional health authorities become outposts of NHS Executive.
	District health authorities and family health service authorities merged to become unified health authorities.
1996	New NHS Complaints Procedure bringing together different procedures and independent review introduced.
1997	**Labour government elected with Tony Blair as Prime Minister.**
	The New NHS: Modern, Dependable – White Paper set out how the internal market would be replaced by a system of 'integrated care', based on partnership and driven by performance as the basis for a ten year programme to renew and improve the NHS.
1998	Review of the Patients Charter and publication of Your Guide to the NHS giving advice to people how to stay healthy and how to use the NHS. Set out what people could do to use the NHS responsibly.
	A First Class Service: Quality in the New NHS – Consultation document setting out strategy for re-organisation of the NHS, proposing setting standards through National Service Frameworks and the National Clinical Institute of Excellence (NICE).
	The *Voluntary Sector Compact* aimed to strengthen partnerships between public services and the voluntary sector and protect their advocacy role.
	Human Rights Act 1998 incorporated the European Convention on Human Rights into UK law and came into force in 2000.
1999	*Saving Lives: Our Healthier Nation* aimed to tackle poor health, particularly for those who are worst off in society. The targets aimed to reduce deaths caused by cancer, coronary heart disease and strokes, accidents and mental illness.
2000	*NHS Plan: a Plan for Investment, a plan for reform* published outlined plans for modernisation of the NHS, including the replacement of CHCs.
	The Local Government Act 2000 separated the executive from the representative role of councillors and set up overview and scrutiny committees to hold health commissioning bodies to account.

User involvement in health – chronology of events – *continued*

Year	Events
2001	*Shifting the Balance of Power within the NHS* – established primary care trusts and reduced Health Authorities from 95 to 28. Replace eight regional offices to four Directorate of Health and Social Care.
	The Bristol Royal Infirmary Inquiry (Kennedy Report) recommended better information and support to patients.
	Health and Social Care Act 2001 introduced a duty to consult on all NHS bodies (Section 11) and a duty on the Secretary of State to provide an independent complaints advocacy services, and enable local authorities to set up health overview and scrutiny committees.
2002	Wanless Report – *Securing Our Future Health* – outlined how money might be saved if people were more engaged in looking after their own health.
	Patient advice and liaison services (PALS) set up.
	Pilot independent complaints advocacy services (ICAS) established.
	NHS and Healthcare Professions Act set up Commission for Patient and Public Involvement in Health and patients' forums and abolished CHCs.
2003	Commission for Patient and Public Involvement in Health begins work.
	Strengthening Accountability, policy and practice guidance for implementation of Section 11 of the Health and Social Care Act published.
	Community health councils are abolished and patient and public involvement forums are established in all NHS trusts.
2004	*Choosing Health: Making Healthier Choices Easier* set out proposals for supporting the public to make healthier and more informed choices.
	Announcement of abolition of Commission for Patient and Public Involvement.
2005	*Together We Can* published by the Home Office as an interdepartmental action plan to strengthen citizens' engagement in delivering local services, covering health, schools, local authorities and the police.

User involvement in health – chronology of events – *continued*

Year	Events
2006	*Our Health, Our Care, Our Say: A New Direction for Community Services* promised patients choice of GP and hospital.
	Power Report published. The independent Power Inquiry was set up by the Joseph Rowntree trusts to look into the problems of the disengagement of citizens in the political process.
	Strong and Prosperous Communities – White Paper gave a stronger role for health services in local area agreements in taking a lead in areas such as mental health with joint budgets and targets agreed at local level.
	Announcement of abolition of patient forums.
	National Health Services Act passed, Section 242 replaced Section 11 of the Health and Social Care Act 2001.
	NHS Centre for Involvement set up (November).
2007	Lyons Inquiry into funding of local government saw a role for local government as 'place shapers' and community leaders.
	Local Government and Public Involvement Act 2007 abolished Commission for Patient and Public Involvement in Health and patients' forums and set up local involvement networks.
2008	Local involvement networks set up and Commission for Patient and Public Involvement in Health and patients forums abolished.

The Story Begins

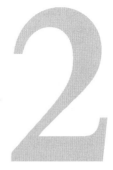

'The people are excluded from forming judgement on various matters of public interest on the ground that expert knowledge is required, and that of course the people cannot possess...The debunking of the expert is an important stage in the history of democratic communities because democracy involves the assertion of the common against the special interest'. Aneurin Bevan, 1938.[1]

Overview

By 1970 it was recognised that the NHS needed reform and it was hoped that increased lay involvement would counter-balance the power of professionals and address inequalities in the NHS.

- The idea of community health councils (CHCs) came from the Conservative Government, but was extended and strengthened by the incoming Labour Government.
- CHCs were seen as a radical new approach that separated representation from management that might be a model for other public services.

It is strange to think that the idea that health services should be designed around the patient is a relatively new one. The first formal recognition that users can help mould health services was in 1974 when CHCs were set up in England and Wales and similar bodies in Scotland and Northern Ireland to represent the interests of local people to managers of the NHS. Until then patients, clients and the public were only considered as recipients of services and their views were not asked or considered important.

Origins of lay involvement

There was a long tradition of volunteers and charitable involvement in providing health and social care (see Box 2.1). Lay people, the great and the good, had been appointed as members of the governing bodies of voluntary hospitals since the opening of St Bartholomew's Hospital in London in 1123 (Peck, 1998). Their main role was to take responsibility for raising funds to maintain the hospital. In contrast local authority-run, poor law hospitals were managed by elected councillors who had an inspection role. In 1948 in setting up hospital management committees, the NHS followed the voluntary hospital model with lay members appointed as supporters rather than inspectors. Though the role was not clearly defined, it was implicit that lay members would combine managerial responsibilities with articulating the interests of the public.

Box 2.1   The voluntary sector and health and social care

In the nineteenth and early twentieth century charities were meeting needs that the state did not, such as healthcare, housing and education. The King's Fund was set up to collect money to support the voluntary hospitals of London in 1897 as the Prince of Wales Hospital Fund for London. In 1911, the gross annual receipts of registered charities exceeded public spending on the Poor Law (Lewis, 1995: 1).

Through **philanthropy** the more fortunate in society offered help to those less fortunate, based on the tradition that status in society also confers duties. For many Victorian middle class women charities were the only available outlet for their energy. However, they were not just rich people giving out charity to the deserving poor; they were also pressure groups for the abolition or promotion of many different causes from temperance to the abolition of child labour and slavery.

Alongside was **mutual aid**, which reacted against the patronage or moral superiority of philanthropy. Through mutual aid members of society help each other on a reciprocal basis, generally the less well off members of society helping their peers. This started spontaneously from groups of men who met regularly and started to put aside a few pence a week for a common purpose. Such groups often provided support for funeral expenses or sickness. From these mutual aid groups arose friendly societies, trade unions, housing associations, people banks and co-operatives (Jones, 2000).

As the state took over more and more services in the twentieth century, the voluntary sector and charities became providers of additional or innovative services. They became increasingly dependent on public funding and employing staff rather than volunteers. Mutual aid was also no longer necessary as the state and labour movement provided the safety net that mutual aid societies had provided before the welfare state.

By the 1960s it was no longer felt that the state could do it all. Cuts in public expenditure meant that volunteers were seen again as a cheaper way of improving public services. The Seebohm report on social work in 1968 saw volunteers working under the direction of paid social workers as a way of expanding services with fewer resources. Though there had been attempts in 1960s to use volunteers in hospitals, there had been opposition because of job insecurity, particularly among nurses. One of the many 'visions' for CHCs was that they would encourage people to volunteer in the NHS.

During the Second World War government took over responsibility for social policy, including the evacuation of children from areas at risk of bombing, rehousing people bombed out of their homes, and providing an emergency medical service. Everyone shared the dangers and the resources through rationing and this gave a new sense of community that led to demands for a more open and egalitarian society. People had not forgotten that the promises made in the First World War to create a land fit for heroes had not been kept. Social rights were a reward for citizens for their duties during the wars and entitled citizens to benefits, such as free healthcare, which were not charity. All political parties realised that plans for a better future were essential for morale and the war effort and so planning for this new society began early in the war. Beveridge published his report in 1942 and from then on there was a consensus about the best way to order a just society and about the relationship of the individual and the state. The consensus about the role of the state and citizens' entitlement to welfare lasted into the 1970s.

The need for reform

The 1960s were a time of change (see Box 2.2). By the late 1960s it was realised that providing for a welfare state was more complex than anticipated. The post-war years were years of central planning. There were concerns from the start that the NHS was a monolithic bureaucracy. Similar concerns were felt about the nationalised industries that included coal, electricity, gas, postal services and transport. These had been created after the Second World War, mainly to protect workers from exploitation. The solution in the nationalised industries had been to set up consultative or consumer councils. However, consumer councils were seen as ineffective (Kelf-Cohen, 1973). They had no contact with the public and so could not represent them. They had limited resources and so relied on management for their information. As a result they were unknown to the public and were not seen as independent.

No similar arrangements had been made for the NHS in 1948, but increased lay involvement came to be seen as a way of addressing some of the problems of the NHS as part of the first reorganisation of the NHS in 1974 since its foundation.

The power of professionals

The NHS before 1974 was configured around hospitals. This was difficult to change because of the power of professionals. As the state took over responsibility for health and welfare, it relied on professionals to deliver these services. Professional power reached its peak with the creation of the NHS in 1948. The power of local government had been reduced with the nationalisation of public utilities and health services. By the middle of the twentieth century professionals had become an exclusive elite protected by their public

---

Box 2.2   The 1960s

The 1960s were a time of innovation and change in British society. There was disillusionment that the welfare state had not yet created utopia.

- The post-war boom had ended. In 1968 sterling was devalued. Economic problems led people to question how much longer universal benefits could be afforded. Prescription charges for medicines had been reintroduced in 1968, having been abolished in 1965.
- Britain was beginning to acknowledge that economic dominance on the global stage was passing to the USA and its empire was crumbling.
- Trade unions were powerful and there were frequent strikes in manufacturing and the public sector.
- In the 1950s and 1960s many immigrants came from India, Pakistan, the West Indies and Africa to work, taking low paid jobs, at the request of government ministers. Until 1962 citizens of the British Commonwealth had the right to come and stay in the UK. The first restrictions on immigration from the British Commonwealth were introduced in 1962. Racial tensions increased and the first Race Relations Acts were passed in 1965 and 1968. Civil rights activists were challenging segregation and discrimination in the USA.
- Women were fighting against discrimination and the Equal Pay Act was passed in 1970. The civil service had just abolished the rule that women must leave on marriage. The contraceptive pill was for the first time enabling women to control their own fertility.
- A new generation of more radical patient and consumer groups were being set up that were questioning traditional ways of providing services and the role of users in them.

---

service ethics (Marquand, 2004). They increasingly saw themselves as specialists with expertise that could not be understood by lay people. Their claim to professional status relied on their technical skills and knowledge which justified their autonomy and clinical freedom. No one but another professional could understand and make judgements on their actions. Patients had few rights at this time. The doctor's duty to do 'good' was seen as more important than the patient's right to information or to make decisions about their own bodies.

However, by the 1960s a new generation of more radical patient and consumer groups and new social movements were emerging and questioning the power of professionals and traditional ways of providing services (see Box 2.3). There was a post-war feeling that the welfare state would continue to expand and that people deserved not just housing, healthcare and subsistence but to be treated with dignity. Just because somebody was in hospital or in need did not mean that they should lose their dignity. People had access to more information and were less deferential. Professional power was now seen as a block to progress. Governments were increasingly frustrated that changes they proposed were blocked by professionals. Though governments

---

Box 2.3   The rise of consumer organisations

By the 1960s new social movements around feminism and anti-racism were emerging. From these came new social welfare movements – around disability rights, older people, race and health. These groups questioned the power of professionals and traditional ways of providing services. It was still a time where there were limited career choices for middle class women and there was a pool of people with time and commitment to be socially innovative.

The women's' movement, working with midwives, campaigned against the medicalisation of childbirth and the increasing use of technology. Doctors had long been competing with midwives, who had traditionally helped women in labour, to control childbirth. Before the NHS most women could not afford a doctor in attendance. With the NHS doctors were able to take over maternity services and reduce the professional independence of midwives. As a result interventions increased and the process of childbirth became medicalised.

New voluntary organisations identified problems that were not generally recognised at the time. Many organisations started when a group of people came together out of self-interest but developed a wider campaigning network, often promoted by socially conscious journalists (Curtis and Sanderson, 2004). Organisations such as Child Poverty Action Group, Pregnancy Advisory Service, Carers UK, Shelter, the National Association for the Welfare of Children in Hospital, the hospice movement, Help the Aged, all started in the 1960s.

There was also a start of shift to user-led organisations. Voluntary organisations run by people affected by the issues, often long-term conditions, wanted to help others often through support groups and helplines and bring about social change as part of the consumer movement. The Claimants Union rebelled against the image of the unemployed as scroungers, the Campaign against Racial Discrimination connected racism with poverty and poor housing. Disabled people questioned the medical model of disability and began to set up organisations that they ran themselves rather than organisations for the benefit of disabled people run by people without disabilities. The Child Poverty Action Group and the Low Pay Unit campaigned to show that poverty had not been defeated by the welfare state. The new groups learnt from the tactics used by the US civil rights movement, in particular the use of the media.

---

controlled the budget, they had no control over clinical decisions and so doctors decided how money was spent. There were also revelations about appalling neglect and abuse in long stay hospitals that raised concerns about whether professionals and lay managers could be trusted to always work in the public interest (see Box 2.4).

Other ways of protecting patients were needed; professionals could no longer be trusted to do this.

Regional inequalities

Though it had been decided to establish a national health service, geographical inequalities and inconsistencies continued. Some regions received

> **Box 2.4   Ely Hospital scandal**
>
> In the late 1960s people had been shocked at the revelations of poor standards of care and even the neglect and abuse of patients in long stay hospitals for people with mental health problems and learning disabilities. In 1969 the Inquiry into Ely Hospital in Cardiff for people with learning disabilities was chaired by a Conservative MP, Geoffrey Howe. It was an indictment of the whole system of long stay institutions for people with mental handicap, describing negligence, brutality and excesses. Revelations showed what could happen when there was no public scrutiny and public trust in professionals was undermined.
>
> Confidence in the system of lay members on boards was also undermined. When the state of the hospital hit the news, the members of the hospital management committee had been more concerned to maintain staff morale than to protect patients from abuse.
>
> The inquiry in Ely had a similar impact on the NHS and public perceptions of professionals as the inquiries into children's cardiac services in Bristol in the 1980s and into the murderous activities of GP, Dr Harold Shipman, in the 1990s.
>
> *Source*: Ely Report (1969) Report of the Committee of Enquiry into Allegations of Ill-treatment of Patients and Other Irregularities at the Ely Hospital, Cardiff. London: HMSO (cmnd 3975).

10 percent more resources and some 10 percent less. London and the South East were considered to be over-resourced, while Wessex, Trent and East Anglia were the poorest (DHSS, 1976a). There was an inequitable allocation of resources between different services. No government initiative seemed able to shift resources from the acute hospital sector to services in the community or long stay hospitals for people with disabilities, mental health problems or learning disabilities.

Unequal access

Those most in need of healthcare are those least likely to receive it – the 'Inverse Care Law' was first articulated by Dr Julian Tudor Hart in 1971. By the 1960s it was realised that providing free health services was not enough. People needed help to make their way through the seemingly inflexible and bureaucratic welfare state. One of the reasons for developing social work as a separate profession in 1968 was to provide a service to act on behalf of those who lacked the knowledge, initiative or energy to act for themselves. This led to the rapid development of social work as a profession in the 1950s and 60s. In 1974 local authorities took over responsibility for social care and social work became an independent profession, rather than under the medical officer of health.

Community involvement had been 'discovered' as a way to tackle deprivation and inequalities in the 1960s. CHCs were seen as a way of providing advocacy at local level for people from deprived communities and for those in neglected long-term care.

The democratic deficit and split of health and social care

When the NHS was established it was not considered politically possible for elected local authorities to manage health services because of concerns about their capacity and the opposition of the medical profession. In 1948 the management of hospitals was taken away from the control of elected local councillors and given to appointed hospital board members. This led to three major problems: a democratic deficit in the NHS where accountability was through the Secretary of State to Parliament; the fragmentation of health and social care; and the marginalisation of public health.

The possibility of transferring the administration of the NHS to local government had been suggested again by a Royal Commission on Local Government in 1969, but was rejected. In the 1974 reforms the NHS took over the running of community health services from local authorities and reduced the number of local government representatives on the new health authorities. Local authorities were not happy about this and, to appease them, they were given control over the appointment of half the CHC membership. It was also seen to add some proxy democratic element to the appointments.

Designing consumer representation

The plans for CHCs evolved in a period of political change with three general elections in four years: Harold Wilson and the Labour Party were defeated by Edward Heath's Conservatives in 1970. In 1973 there was an oil crisis caused by a sudden price increase by the Middle Eastern oil producers in retaliation for the support of the West for Israel in the Yom Kippur War. In the UK the cost of living rose by 10 percent in a single year and the gross domestic product was reduced by 5 percent. The oil crisis and industrial unrest, in particular the miners strike, led Heath to call an election in November 1973 to assert his power over the trade unions with the slogan 'Who Governs Britain?' The electorate's answer was the Labour Party and Harold Wilson returned but with no overall majority. A further election was called in February 1974 which gave Harold Wilson a tiny but overall majority. A further election in October 1974 gave the Labour Government a bigger majority.

The Conservative vision

There was all-party agreement that the NHS needed reform. The Labour Government had outlined plans in 1970 for district committees made up of a chairman with half the members appointed by and drawn from the proposed new area health authorities (AHAs) and the other half drawn from people living or working in the district. Their purpose was to supervise the running of services and to serve as one of the channels through which local people could keep the area health authority informed of any problems they encountered with local health services (DHSS, 1970). They were to have no separate budget and no statutory powers.

Box 2.5   Separating representation and management

The separation of the functions of management and representation had long been a debate among local authorities. In 1967 the Maud Report on local authorities recommended that there should be a small management group of councillors responsible for decisions and supervising the work of the officers. The rest of the councillors would sit on committees which were not directing or controlling bodies but would, among other duties consider the interests, reactions and criticisms of the public and convey them to the officers and, if necessary, to the management board. This model was rejected by local authorities. However, a similar structure emerged over 30 years later with the introduction of 'cabinet' government in local authorities in the Local Government Act 2000.

In setting up CHCs the incoming Labour Government did not accept that it was possible or desirable to make a clear-cut distinction between management of public services and representation of consumer interests. '*Our whole national democratic process as it has involved over the years is a complex interweave of management and representation*' (DHSS, 1974a: 5). It was proposed that CHC members could also be AHA members and that NHS employees or family practitioners could be eligible to serve on CHCs. It also proposed that CHCs should be able to elect two members, one of whom should be a local authority councillor, to be appointed by the RHA to serve for two years as a member of the matching AHA (or four members in single district areas).

However, these proposals were not pursued. Similar ideas re-emerged in debates 30 years later over the replacement of CHCs, where the Government wanted patient and public involvement forums to have the right to elect one of their members as a non-executive director on trust boards. This proposal was also not pursued.

The Conservatives when they came into government later that year felt that Labour's proposals would lead to a dangerous confusion between management on the one hand and the community's reaction to management on the other (see Box 2.5). They wanted members of the new authorities to be chosen for their personal qualities, and not as representatives of either local authorities or health professions. Clearly this made sense in terms of upward accountability but was not compatible with accountability to local communities or professional peers.

In May 1971 it was proposed in a consultative document that managerial ability would be the main criterion for the selection of new health authority members. The idea for a separate consumer body called a community health council came from the Conservative Government when Keith Joseph was Minister of Health. The idea suggested itself in the words of one of the ministers involved, '*as soon as we had decided to go for unrepresentative [area health authorities]*' (Klein and Lewis, 1976: 13). The White Paper proposed that the new AHAs would set up a CHC for each district as it was '*important to have more representational mechanisms by which local attitudes can be known and safeguards built in*' (DHSS, 1971: para 20). CHCs would have the right to be consulted and to visit NHS premises and a duty to produce an annual report.

Members of AHAs were to manage while members of CHCs were to represent the views of the consumer. CHCs were also seen as a way of encouraging co-operation between health and personal social services by involving the local community in the NHS. Indeed some of the early discussions about CHCs took place at the Department of Health and Social Security (DHSS) in the context of how to integrate services at local level, not about consumer representation. Opinion within the DHSS was not unanimous about the wisdom of setting up CHCs as independent, non-executive bodies. In the discussions at the Department, there were some who were worried lest CHCs – without any direct responsibilities – would become 'naggers and stirrers-up of complaints'. Others simply thought that CHCs would be ineffective.

Parliament was concerned about the decline in local authority members and the loss of the democratic element in the NHS. A number of significant changes were made in response to backbench prodding in the Lords and Commons. Initially the proposal was that half CHC members were to be appointed by local authorities and half by the local NHS management. As a member of the House of Lords observed in the debate: *'The game keeper has been told to appoint his own poachers and nobody believes it will work'* (Webster, 1996: 517). Under pressure from the Government's own supporters as well as from the opposition, the membership was changed to half nominated by local authorities, one-third elected by voluntary organisations and one-sixth selected by regional health authorities (RHAs). Greater independence was given to CHCs with responsibility for financing and accommodating CHCs transferred from the area level to the more distant RHAs. There was further support for more independence for CHCs from the Davies Committee that had been set up after the Ely Inquiry to look at developing a national complaints procedure for the NHS. In an interim report the Committee saw an active role for CHCs in helping complainants and recommended strengthening their independence to enable them to do this (Webster, 1996).

Klein and Lewis (1976: 16) point out that the reason why ministers were prepared to change the original Bill in response to backbench pressure was that CHCs were peripheral to the reforms. A minister is quoted as saying: '(We) *had no fixed ideas about how they should be constituted or how they should work. We were much happier to make concessions on this part of the Bill than on the management structure. And it always helps politically to be able to make some concessions'*.

The Labour vision

The Labour Government came back into office on 5 March 1974. It was too late to halt the NHS Reorganisation Act 1973 which was due to come into force on 1 April (see Box 2.6). CHCs were set up in each district to represent the interest of local people to managers of the NHS.

The new Labour Government saw the possibilities in the Conservative vision for CHCs and set about strengthening them. Dr David Owen, the new

---

Box 2.6   The NHS Reorganisation Act 1973

The Act set up 90 area health authorities in England who were responsible for planning, management and developing services jointly with their matching local authorities. Members were appointed by the local authority, the professions and by the Secretary of State.

- Area health authorities (AHAs) were accountable to 14 regional health authorities (RHAs) who were accountable to the Secretary of State.
- Alongside each AHA was a family practitioner committee (FPC) which administered the contracts of GPs, dentists, pharmacists and opticians.
- Most areas were split into health districts, each of which was administered by a district management team (DMT).

This replaced a more fragmented system where local authorities managed community health services; executive councils administered family practitioner services, boards of governors managed the old voluntary hospitals which were the elite training and specialist hospitals; and regional hospital boards managed the vast majority of hospitals that had been under local authority control before 1948. All were accountable directly to the Ministry of Health.

Source: NHS Reorganisation Act 1973.

Minister of Health, saw CHCs as a catalyst for change. They could take on the professions in a way that Government could not: '*It is the pressure as much as political leadership which is needed to ensure the ultimate abolition of the present inequalities in health care provision*' (Owen, 1976: 60). Similar thinking led to the Government to fund national pressure groups such as MIND for mental health services and MENCAP for people with learning disabilities.

In April the Labour Government published a White Paper that proposed changes that strengthened the independence and rights of CHCs: staff posts were opened up to external applicants through open competition; spokesmen for the district management team were required to attend CHC meetings when invited; CHCs had the right to be consulted by RHAs as well as AHAs. They also did not accept the clear-cut distinction between management of public services and representation of consumer interests (see Box 2.5).

The role originally planned for CHCs also grew. A minister involved is quoted as saying: '*we first decided that there should be such a body and then decided what it should do. As we worked on the CHCs, we found more things for them to do*' (Klein and Lewis, 1976: 15). The statutory duties of CHCs were broad. They were to keep under review the operation of the health service in its district and make recommendations as to the improvement of that service and to publish an annual report. There was no guidance on how CHCs should perform these duties. The list of 'matters to which community health councils might wish to direct their attention' published by the DHSS was ambitious. It included: the effectiveness of services, the planning of services; collaboration between health services and local authorities; assessing the extent to which district health facilities conformed to those published in the departmental policies; the share of available resources devoted to the care of long stay patients unable to protect their own interests; facilities; waiting periods; quality of catering; and monitoring the volume and type of complaints received about the service or institution (DHSS, 1974b).

The rights and duties of CHCs were also strengthened and they were given statutory powers to obtain information, visit hospitals and other institutions and access to health authorities and their senior officers. The DHSS advised AHAs to allow a CHC representative to attend AHA meetings with the right to speak but not to vote. They could attend family practitioner committee (FPC) meetings, as observers, at the discretion of individual FPCs.

A major new power was given to CHCs by the incoming Labour Government. If the CHC agreed to a hospital closure, it was no longer necessary to seek the approval of the Secretary of State for the closure. This gave NHS managers an incentive to consult CHCs about hospital closures and avoid the long delays involved in seeking DHSS approval. However, CHCs which objected to closures were expected to make a detailed constructive counter-proposal that took account of the factors, including restraints on resources, which led the health authority to propose the closure. This expected CHCs to take on a management role in making these counter-proposals, hardly realistic given their resources and was not compatible with their role as community representatives.

A national council funded by central government was proposed to advise and assist CHCs. '*It believes that such a body could make a vital contribution towards enabling the CHCs effectively to fulfil their role as the local representatives of the users of health services. It would provide a national voice for CHCs; it could, for example, arrange conferences for members and staff of CHCs, promote and if necessary finance research into methods of ascertaining the views of users of the health services, and undertake or arrange surveys of user opinion on behalf of CHCs*' (DHSS, 1974a: 11).

Rudolf Klein and Janet Lewis concluded that: '*Community Health Councils were invented almost by accident because, when the plans for a reorganised health service were almost complete, all those involved realised that something was missing: an element which could be presented and seen as providing a degree of local democracy, consumer participation or public involvement in the affairs of the NHS. Effectively CHCs were therefore invented to fill a political vacuum, and their subsequent evolution and the uncertainties about their role reflect their improvised beginning*' (1976: 11).

Setting up the councils

The Minister, David Owen, appointed two ministerial advisers, Lady Mary Marre and Councillor Ken Collis, to advise him on the process of setting up CHCs and in particular to find out the views of CHCs on what they wanted and what they needed to carry out the duties laid down for them. They reported to Ministers in March 1975 (Gerrard, 2006, Appendix 1).

RHAs in England and the Welsh Office in Wales were the establishing bodies for CHCs, with delegated authority from the Secretary of State. The functions that RHAs performed for CHCs included: the appointment of members to CHCs; determining CHC staff levels and employing staff; administering arrangements for office accommodation and services; determining CHC budgets and monitoring expenditure; and considering appeals in disputes between CHCs and AHAs.

The establishment and oversight of 207 CHCs was delegated to RHAs so that CHCs could be clearly seen to be independent of AHAs who were not responsible for allocating resources or involved in staff appointments. Neither the DHSS nor the RHA had the authority to give directions to CHCs apart from financial arrangements. The attitude of RHAs has been described as *'benevolent if somewhat headmasterly'* (Gerrard, 2006: 75). Sometimes RHAs tried to restrict CHC activities, with little success but leading to conflict and disputes in some regions. At this time generally ministers supported CHCs in asserting their independence against RHAs.

Guidance to RHAs was published in January 1974 and RHAs were expected to set up CHCs by April. Not surprisingly it took longer than this. There were great variations in how RHAs set about the task. Some were directive, some more consultative and one (the West Midlands) was dilatory because of its hostility to the idea of CHCs (Gerrard, 2006). However, most CHCs had held their first meetings by September 1974.

RHAs decided how many members each CHC would have and this varied between 22 and 33 members. Half were appointed by local authorities, one-third elected by voluntary organisation and the remainder by RHAs (see Box 2.7). The ministerial advisers pointed to the wide differences in how RHAs interpreted the guidance: some CHCs had a disproportionate number of members living outside the district and some people were members of more than one community health council. Appointments were for four years and members could serve two terms. The appointing body could be asked to replace a member if they did not attend meetings for six months. In the first year some members resigned. According to Jack Hallas (1976) the drop out rate was about 12½ percent in the first year. A number of members became disenchanted with the prospect of a do-it-yourself council, particularly those with a local authority background. In Oxfordshire ten out of 30 CHC members resigned in the first year, eight being local authority nominees. In many areas the attendance record of local authority nominees was much lower than other nominees. CHCs from the start did not accept inactive members. They tended to enforce the six month expulsion rule rigorously, indicating a confidence that more appropriate replacements would be found. In second round appointments in the Yorkshire Region where there were 150 places in 17 CHCs for voluntary organisations, there were more than 1000 requests from voluntary bodies to be considered for representation (Hallas, 1976).

Each CHC had an overall budget allocated by the regional health authority based on a population as well as a negotiated amount for staff, rent and other

---

Box 2.7   Appointments to CHCs

Local authorities appointed half the members. They were more likely to hold other public appointments than members appointed by other routes. Four out of five were members of one of the three main political parties. Of the total CHC membership almost one-third belonged to the Labour Party and one-sixth to the Conservative Party. Over four-fifths of members nominated by local authorities were councillors.

Voluntary organisations elected one-third of members. Regional health authorities were expected to draw up the list of voluntary organisations eligible to put forward nominations and to vote. Some regions restricted eligibility to organisations related to health, others accepted any voluntary organisation with an interest in the area. The object was to bias selection deliberately to ensure representation by proxy of the most vulnerable sections of the community whose voices were rarely heard.

The National Council for Social Service provided guidance to local voluntary organisations on how they might set about choosing their share of CHC members. It suggested that CHC members should be selected by constituencies, each of whom would represent a particular group of users: children, elderly, mentally ill or handicapped, physically handicapped and a general category. This ensured the representation of specific and particularly vulnerable care groups. One in ten CHC members was a member of an organisation concerned with mental health, while one quarter was from organisations concerned with the elderly. Almost two-fifths of CHC members were members of voluntary organisations concerned with health or social care and most of them were officeholders in those organisations. Organisations concerned with immigrants were given particular attention in guidance given to RHAs. One out of every 20 CHC members was a member of such organisations. Without voluntary organisation representatives, the representation for these groups would have been more than halved.

One-sixth of members were appointed by RHAs. This was to provide a role for hospital management committee members who had lost their places and to ensure that some CHC members knew about health services. Apart from appointing men and women with previous health service experience, appointments were also to include representatives of bodies, such as women's organisations, trade unions, the churches and the immigrant bodies that might not otherwise be appointed. RHA appointees were largely drawn from people who were already involved in public committees and were of higher social class. Klein and Lewis concluded that there was no evidence that RHA nominees contributed a distinctive style to CHCs activities.

Source: Klein and Lewis, 1976.

---

expenditure. There were wide discrepancies between RHAs. For example, the allocation to CHCs per head of population was 11.6 pence in South West Thames compared to 5.7 pence in Wessex.[2] These regional discrepancies were never addressed and continued into the 1990s. Hallas (1976), as well as the Ministerial Advisers, identified frugality as a feature of all CHCs. From the earliest days CHCs were concerned to be seen by the public as careful spenders of money. This meant that some stayed in hospital premises at the cost of a perceived loss of independence. Others were reluctant to pay the costs of staff or members to go to conferences.

The way of appointing CHC members led to variations that reflected the local area (see Box 2.8). CHCs were required to elect the chair from among their number. Before the secretaries were appointed, chairs set a style for the CHC. This depended on the background of chair. Local authority appointees tended to be businesslike and focussed, while chairs from the voluntary sector tended to be more diffuse and deliberative. Chairs from a hospital management background tended to see role of the CHC as about hospitals not health (Hallas, 1976). The profile of CHC chairs was different from that of the rest of the membership: they were more likely to be men and local authority appointees, or nominated by RHAs. They were more likely to be magistrates or school governors than the average CHC member. One-third had a university degree compared to one-fifth of all CHC members (Klein and Lewis, 1976).

The selection of staff was the choice of each CHC. Most CHCs had an establishment of two full time staff. It had been expected that most CHC secretaries (later called chief officers) would come from an NHS background. However, secretaries came from a variety of backgrounds, just under half

---

Box 2.8　The first CHC members

A national survey of CHC members in England and Wales and provided a snapshot of membership at the time of their appointment. The survey found that members tended to be older, male and more middle class than the general population. However, they also had far more than their share of non-manual workers such as clerks, salesmen and draughtsman and 15 percent of members were manual workers. When membership profiles were broken down by region and by district a varied picture emerged, reflecting the social and political culture of specific communities. For example, CHCs in the North West Thames region had an above average proportion of CHC members who were women, under 35, in social classes one and two, who went to a public school and had a university degree. In contrast the Welsh CHC members were consistently below the national average on all these counts. In looking at individual districts the study found that CHCs reflected the community which they represented, though not in a precise statistical sense. Though this snapshot was for the members in the first round of appointments, a survey in 1982 in South West Thames region found little change in the profile of membership (University of Surrey, 1982).

Klein and Lewis concluded that a variety of methods had created a greater diversity among members – with a wider representation of social experience, occupational background, interest groups and public service and know-how than might otherwise have been the case. It was also likely to lead to variations in the ethos and approaches of individual CHCs.

Source: Klein and Lewis, 1976.

from the NHS but others from the voluntary sector, local government, the armed forces and the private sector. Those involved in the initial training for CHC staff reported that the *'enthusiasm and initiative of Secretaries was far higher than expected by those used to training NHS managers'* (Hallas, 1976: 14). Once appointed the secretary was influential. The malleability of the job was such that it could be shaped around the interests of the incumbent.

The new CHC also had to decide what sort of office it wanted. Many felt that CHC premises needed to be outside the NHS in order to establish the CHC's independence from the NHS. Shop front premises were seen as a way of raising the public profile of the CHC and make it accessible to the public, though these were expensive to rent and some RHAs would not pay. One in five CHCs were in shop front premises and about 12 percent in hospitals or other NHS buildings (Farrell and Adams, 1981). The Royal Commission (1979) recommended that health authorities should encourage all CHCs to find high street or easily accessible premises wherever possible. The choice of office had implications for the work of the CHC. Offices that were easily accessible to the public tended to attract more 'customers' looking for information and advice, often on issues unrelated to the NHS or health. This could take up a lot of staff time and distract them from other activities. This became important in the debates in the 1990s about the most appropriate focus for CHCs within their limited resources. Was it visibility in the community or was it more important for the CHC to work more closely and be more allied to the NHS?

Scotland and Northern Ireland

The NHS Reorganisation Act 1973 covered England and Wales and there was separate legislation for Scotland and Northern Ireland. Local Health Councils were set up in Scotland as the equivalent of CHCs. In Northern Ireland combined health and social services boards were set up that dealt directly with the Northern Ireland Office, with a committee equivalent to the CHC for each administrative district. They were not as independent as CHCs. NHS bodies appointed members and they had no right to attend health board meetings. As a late amendment local health councils in Scotland were given the right to select their own chair (Webster, 1996: 55).

Conclusions

Many different expectations were piled onto CHCs from the start in an attempt to address the faultlines that had emerged in the structure of the NHS. The author was among the CHC secretaries appointed in 1974. Strangely though the many different expectations were demanding and unrealistic, they were also liberating. CHCs had the freedom to develop in different ways. Most NHS managers were unfamiliar with their communities and with consumerism, CHCs had something new and different to bring to the NHS.

They were exciting times. Those of us involved in the first CHCs knew we had something to prove. We felt we were embarking on a new path which would provide an example to other public services of how they could relate to their users and communities.

Community Health Councils – The Rise 1974–1979

3

'*In a sense we, in the NHS, fell into the sin of overweening pride. [Community Health] Councils can help the service recapture some of the dream of Aneurin Bevan which, because of our fall from economic grace, now has more potential for realisation than at any time since the late 1940s*'. Jack Hallas, 1976: 65.

Overview

This chapter outlines how CHCs developed their role in the 1970s.

■ There were many expectations of CHCs, but no clear view of their role or guidance on how they should work.

■ This led to wide variations in what CHCs did, how they interpreted their role and to disputes between CHCs and managers.

■ In the first few years CHCs were largely seen as a success and the verdict of the Royal Commission was that CHCs should be strengthened.

■ The way CHCs were set up made it hard for a national movement to develop and for them to adapt to meet the challenges of the 1980s and 1990s.

Introduction

Community health councils (CHCs) had their roots in the 1960s – a time of innovation and hope founded in a belief in the welfare state and social rights. This was quickly followed by the crises of the 1970s. When CHCs started there was economic stagnation. Inflation in 1975 was 25 percent. In 1976 the Labour Government was forced to go to the International Monetary Fund for a loan, which was given, provided that public sector expenditure was reduced. As a result there was wage restraint and industrial unrest. There were strikes and breakdown in public services. A strike of grave diggers meant that funerals were delayed for weeks. Rubbish piled up in the streets. The Labour Party was divided by battles with the militant left wing. Many of the right wing leaders in the end left the Labour Party to form the Social

Democratic Party in 1981. The 1974 management reorganisation was disruptive for the NHS. Klein (2001) describes the time as the politics of disillusionment that led to the setting up of the Royal Commission in 1977 – as a way of deferring dealing with the problems that beset the NHS following the 1974 reorganisation.

CHCs were a radical and innovative idea and no one knew in 1974 how they would turn out. There was considerable apprehension on the part of managers and professionals on what they might do and how they might be controlled. On the one hand they feared that CHCs would be troublemakers, adding to the problems of the NHS and encouraging complaints. On the other; they feared that CHCs would be 'lap dogs' to the NHS and not use their independent voice. Would CHC members see their first loyalty to the NHS or would they speak up on behalf of local people? In these early days there was a lot of interest in the CHC experiment. It was not often that governments invented new institutions, which offered academics an opportunity to study their evolution. For researchers, such as Klein and Lewis (1976), it was interesting to see whether central accountability and planning could be reconciled with responsiveness to consumer views at local level. There was also interest in whether CHCs, that split consumer representation from management, could provide a model for more widespread use in public services in Britain and elsewhere. Training was provided by the King's Fund, the Nuffield Centre in Leeds and Manchester University for staff and members. Later the School of Advanced Urban Studies, Bristol University, ran training courses for CHC staff and produced a handbook for CHC members. These were led by Chris Ham, later adviser to the Department of Health.

What CHCs did

CHCs may have started out as a symbolic gesture to participation and democracy, but they soon took on a life of their own way beyond that intended. It was a time of enthusiasm and innovation. With little guidance and a wide remit, CHCs had a blank canvass (see Box 3.1). Looking at the annual reports for the first year of CHCs the amount of work and diversity of activities that were undertaken in that time is striking. All commentators observed the diversity among CHCs from the earliest days. They joined planning teams, responded to consultations, made counter-proposals and carried out surveys (see Chapter 5). CHCs offered information advice to the public and assisted complainants (see Chapter 6). They carried out health education and health promotion (see Chapter 7).

Jack Hallas (1976) undertook a survey based on visits to CHCs in the Yorkshire Region, where he reported that there were dramatic differences, often sharp enough to make the observer despair of finding any common denominators. He did, however, identify common themes. As well as frugality and a strong sense of loyalty to their districts, he observed that CHCs were insular and reluctant to take up experiments from other councils or learn from them. In spite of all the differences, however, CHCs shared the

---

Box 3.1   Expectations of CHCs

The Labour Government in the early days had many different expectations of CHCs. They wanted CHCs to:

- Strengthen democracy in the health service, and to take on professionals and help implement national policies at local level.
- Encourage people to take up vaccination and screening programmes.
- Get involved in planning and also work with health authorities about alternative services involving closures, taking a deliberative rather than populist view of services.
- Get involved in local debates about fluoridation of the water supplies and road safety.
- Help the interface of health and social care between NHS and local authorities.
- Have shop front premises so that the public could call on the CHC for information and advice and assistance in making complaints.
- Promote volunteering and encourage people to volunteer in the NHS.

---

same priorities – a concern for primary and community services, mental health, mental handicap, the elderly and children.

How CHCs worked

Each CHC had its own ways of working. Generally the CHC and its work were managed by a triumvirate of the secretary, chair and vice chair who oversaw the work and co-ordinated the working groups. The guidance to CHCs had suggested that they might set up working groups and from the start most work was carried out in working groups and not in the main CHC meetings. The most important role of the secretary was in providing administrative support for working groups. Mostly planning teams were set up for client groups, such as mental illness, the elderly and children that reflected the areas covered by district healthcare planning teams. This model was suited to urban but not to rural areas, where geographical committees were often more appropriate. There were debates among CHCs about much time they should devote to planning which was unlikely to lead to short-term changes or results for local people (Hallas, 1976).

As time went on the perception of members of their role changed. The Ministerial Advisers on CHCs noted that initially many members saw it as another outside committee which only involved interest and attendance at meetings. As the first year of work progressed, the desire of CHC members to make a contribution to NHS thinking, their appreciation of the need for training, and work outside council meetings meant that CHC membership involved considerable commitment of time and energy (Dunford, 1977). The way the CHC defined its role and the relationship between staff and members affected the commitment required of members. If the CHC was member-led, seeing the secretary as an administrator, it was up to members to generate

---

Box 3.2   Commitment of CHC members

As a general rule less than half the members were actively involved and so the work-load fell unevenly on members (Levitt, 1980).

The time given to the CHC by members was considerable. In a survey of the South West Thames region in 1982, 38 percent of members said they gave between three to five hours a week and 14 percent gave six or more hours a week.

Representatives of voluntary organisations gave more time to the work of the CHC than members appointed by local authorities or the RHA. This was also reflected in attendance at CHC meetings. Half of voluntary organisation representatives attended more than 90 percent of the meetings, in comparison to 25 percent of local authority appointees and 35 percent of RHA appointees (University of Surrey, 1982).

This pattern continued into the 1990s and CHC members remained a formidable volunteer force to the end. A survey of members in 1995 found that just under half of members stated that CHC work was taking an average of around four to six hours a week, 21 percent claimed that CHC work takes between 8–12 hours a week. The authors concluded that the figures indicated a workforce of volunteers averaging nearly 3000 hours a week on CHC duties or 100,000 hours a year working for the NHS without pay (Arnold et al., 1995a).

---

new ideas and explore new areas of work. Because most CHCs saw themselves as generating their own information, this imposed a much greater burden on members than if they had merely acted as part of ongoing communication networks (see Box 3.2). Farrell and Adams (1981) found that the number of surveys and projects that the CHC undertook was directly related to the number of active CHC members. There was therefore a case for increasing the number of members on the CHC rather than reducing them. One-third of CHCs also had used work experience and job creation schemes that aimed to give young people work experience and new skills.

The regulations allowed for one-third of the people serving on CHC committees to be co-opted. For CHCs this was a way of strengthening themselves with additional volunteers. People co-opted onto committees were able to participate fully in the activities of CHCs, but were not permitted to vote at meetings. Many CHCs used co-options to get additional experience or skills to work on particular areas or services and also to meet any gaps in the membership. Some people were interested in promoting particular services, such as maternity services or mental health, but not in the wider collective responsibilities of being a CHC member. By 1980 62 percent of CHCs had co-opted members (Farrell and Adams, 1981). This also continued in the mid-1990s; there were many co-opted members involved in the work of CHCs. The number of co-opted members per region varied from 17 in Trent to 163 in South Thames (Insight, 1996).

The few studies that have been carried out found that the most important factor in influencing the effectiveness of the CHC was the staff (Hallas, 1976;

Klein and Lewis, 1976; Moon and Lupton, 1995). A survey in 1985 asked CHC secretaries and district general managers what they considered the most important factors influencing the effectiveness of a CHC. Both general managers and CHC secretaries considered that the secretary was the most important factor (Hogg, 1986).

Regional associations

CHCs were essentially local bodies. They identified with their own locality and often supported the district management team at area, regional and national level. Individual CHCs orchestrated campaigns on regional and national issues (see Box 3.3). From an early stage there were regional meetings of CHCs. These were useful for regional health authority officers, who could use them to communicate with CHCs in the region. Jack Hallas (1976) noted that early on CHCs made alliances with the regional tier rather than area health authorities. The organisation of CHCs in the regions was generally loose, supported by CHC staff and most had no dedicated workers. Regional health authority boundaries included inner and outer city as well as rural areas and there were conflicts between their interests, particularly around resource allocation as well as different political allegiances between urban and rural CHCs.

At this time there were systematic attempts to redistribute resources to have a fairer distribution between the regions which was also divisive. In 1976 the report of the Resource Allocation Working Party (RAWP) was published which recommended that resources for hospital and community services should be allocated on the basis on the population (DHSS, 1976a). The reallocation of resources between regions under RAWP meant that some areas gained and others lost. This redistribution was meant to be achieved

---

Box 3.3   CHC campaigns

CHCs worked together within and between regions.

- In September 1977 the West Midlands RHA dropped its plan to close St Wulston's Hospital, a specialist schizophrenia unit which offered a regional service, following a campaign by West Midlands CHCs and co-ordinated by their regional association.
- Brent CHC along with 11 other CHCs campaigned about DepoProvera, a contraceptive, given by injection mainly to Black and Asian women and not licensed for long-term use.
- In Wales Merthyr and Cynon Valley CHC launched a national campaign for people who had suffered side effects of the heart drug Eraldin. Astonishingly, at that time patients did not have the right to know whether or not they had been prescribed the drug, if their GP chose not to tell them.

Sources: CHC News, October, No 24, 1977: No 32, June 1978.

out of new money, but it led to cuts in losing areas, particularly London. London had poor community and primary care services and CHCs wanted improvements rather than cuts. CHCs fought for their local interests and added to the difficulties in implementation.

CHCs at national level

CHC News

The Government demonstrated its commitment to CHCs from the beginning. In May 1975 the DHSS had funded the first issue of CHC News, a magazine for CHCs with aspirations to a wider audience. The DHSS provided a grant to produce CHC News and provide an information service. The remaining funding was to come from membership subscriptions. CHC News was published monthly, initially by a team based at the King's Fund until it was taken over by the Association of CHCs for England and Wales. It was source of strength for CHCs and a convincing advertisement for them as it was widely distributed in the DHSS, professional and academic circles as well as the health press and medical journals. It subscribed to a press cuttings service which provided daily news on CHCs in the national and local press.

Planning the national body

The NHS Reorganisation Act 1973 included provision for a national organisation to advise and assist CHCs in performing their functions, but did not bind the Secretary of State to set up one up. In February 1975 the Nuffield Centre for Health Service Studies held a Conference in London for CHCs. At the conference Dr David Owen, Minister of State for Health, announced his intention to form a steering committee, which would prepare proposals for the establishment of a national council for CHCs. He hoped that it would be set up by the end of 1975. He wanted the council to present a strong independent patients' voice at national level. He thought this was what CHCs wanted and that it could address some of the difficulties CHCs were experiencing in the co-operation they received from the NHS, in particular from family practitioner committees. The Government saw CHCs as an important supporter in implementing polices at local level. Hallas noted that: '*He gave the impression that this centrally collected information could become a powerful aid to a minister in helping to put to right some of the unfortunate administrative features of the reorganised NHS*' (Hallas, 1976: 11).

A steering group was set up to advise on the national organisation with the costs met by the King's Fund. It was made up of representatives from the regions. However, things did not go as the government planned. The steering group met opposition and had to proceed carefully. From the start many CHCs resented the idea of a national body being imposed on them and they mistrusted the Government's motives. The Conservative Party in opposition tabled a motion seeking to get the regulations that set up the national association annulled.[1] The controversy over whether or not there should be a national association was fuelled partly by the early success of regional arrangements in various parts of the country, which meant that a national association was seen as less important. Each CHC had its own style and many were ambivalent about involvement on a regional, let alone a national level. There was no longer talk of a national council, but an association. The steering group considered whether the national body should be able to evaluate CHCs but resisted any proposal, which would be seen as an inspectorate. Following consultation the steering group supported the concept of a much looser confederation of councils, having a small unit working directly to them rather than being seen as a permanent secretariat looking to the DHSS (Hallas, 1976).

There was also controversy about whether or not staff should be included in the new association. Some members felt secretaries were becoming too powerful, while some secretaries were wary of being seen as mere committee secretaries. Some of this concern arose from the fact that CHC staff had set up their own association, the Society of CHC Secretaries, in 1975 to act as a professional organisation. While most CHCs found ways of working together, whether CHCs should be led by members or by staff was a recurrent theme in the politics of the Association of Community Health Councils for England and Wales (ACHCEW). This resonated in the establishment of PPI forums as member-led organisations and this justified the limited staff resources that were made available to them (see Chapter 9).

Setting up the association

A conference was held in autumn 1976. This decided in favour of forming an association. One hundred and twelve CHCs voted in favour, 91 against and 26 did not attend the conference. The aims of the new national association were to provide a forum to CHCs, to act as their national voice, to provide information and advisory services and to encourage, promote and protect the independence of individual CHCs.

The national association had not started well with many CHCs opposing its formation. At the time of the first annual general meeting in 1977 over a quarter of CHCs (63 out of 229) decided not to join, though the subscription did not come from their budget. ACHCEW at the start set about wooing individual CHCs whose support it could not take for granted if it was to survive. The lack of support also meant that the regional associations did not provide an infrastructure for ACHCEW that would have strengthened its links to individual CHCs and provided a means of accountability and dissemination. ACHCEW also set about building bridges at national level with NHS and professional bodies. Mike Gerrard (2006), the first director of ACHCEW, concludes that this was worthwhile so that by the time the first attempt to abolish CHCs was made in 1980 there were sufficient positive relationships to ensure formidable support for CHCs.

As CHCs gained in confidence, they began to question government policy, causing increasing concerns in Whitehall. CHCs were supposed to be promoting the implementation of policy – not questioning it. CHC News was forthright in its criticisms of government policy. CHCs were discovering, as community workers had before, that many of the problems of disadvantaged communities could not be solved by better health services, but needed more radical solutions involving jobs and income.

Emerging tensions

However, after six years, some of the flaws and the tensions that led to the decline of CHCs in the 1980s were also evident. There were debates about CHCs and their future at this time: the purpose of CHCs and relationships with management. Debates about accountability followed later. These debates persisted throughout the life of CHCs and still continue with successor organisations. CHCs were set up as autonomous local bodies and this led to internal conflicts and limited their ability to develop as a movement and adapt to the changing world.

What were CHCs for?

There were different visions for CHCs from the start. The original Conservative vision was of the CHC as a local consumer group, who would make representations to health authorities on behalf of local residents about detailed aspects of the local delivery of services. They did not want CHCs to be independent, become involved in policy or be in any way political. The Labour vision was more ambitious.

No organisation with an average of two members of staff and a group of volunteers could meet the expectations laid on CHCs. Each CHC had to find its own way. First, how far should CHCs promote or provide services? Some CHCs became involved, often with voluntary groups, in providing a patient advocacy services, information, training and health promotion. Others considered that CHCs should press the NHS to provide such services if they were needed, rather than directly providing them.

Second, should CHCs cover the NHS or the wider community? Some CHCs restricted their comments to services provided by the health authority. Others took a broad view of their remit to include public health and care for vulnerable groups of patients in social care where they considered there was a gap, such as monitoring local social services, environmental hazards, or homeless people in bed and breakfast accommodation who were not otherwise represented.

Third, should CHCs choose priorities for the community? Some CHCs put forward the views of the community, without choosing priorities, which they considered to be the task of management. Others felt that, by assisting management in choosing priorities, they were actively helping to put more resources into services for priority groups, such as mentally ill, handicapped and elderly people.

Fourth, should CHCs react to the NHS or set the agenda? It was easy for a CHC to find that all their time was taken up responding to tasks given to them by NHS managers. Some CHCs decided to concentrate their energies in areas where they felt that they might have more impact and gave priority to identifying unmet needs and working with the community to promote good practices.

Fifth, what should the central activities of the CHC be? CHCs concentrated on different activities. Some, generally those with high street premises, gave priority to dealing with individuals and their problems. Others affected by NHS cuts gave priority to responding to consultation documents on closures and changes of use. Others looked out to the community and tried to set an agenda for health services in their area.

Many CHCs were uneasy about the eclectic and the idiosyncratic ways that some CHCs developed. One member commented: '*CHC News induces a sense of inferiority in many CHC members and secretaries when they read of the many and varied activities of their colleagues up and down the country.... It is only when the projects are analysed that the doubts appear. It is not the function of a CHC to run the health education department or a citizens advice bureau... There is scarcely anything in everyday life which does not have a bearing on health. That a CHC should therefore be prepared to concern itself with every aspect of everyday life does not necessarily follow. There are two important areas, of social services and environmental health, into which many CHCs have strayed and that exceeded their terms of reference*'.[2]

Philip Hunt was appointed a CHC Secretary in London in 1974. Later, as a Minister in the House of Lords, he was involved in the abolition of CHCs. In 2006 he reflected on this experience: '*CHCs were a great idea in 1974. It was a great job at the beginning and many staff wanted to be involved as it was new. I came from the NHS to be secretary of a CHC, but we seemed to be shadowing the health authority all the time. What we did was dominated by the producers, and by special interests, such as maternity, elderly, children and mental health. The membership was skewed to selected voluntary organisations and this dominated what CHCs did. We did not really understand what consumerism was*' (Hogg, 2006a).

So perhaps the first source of decline was unrealistic and, perhaps, incompatible expectations. Everyone acknowledged that some CHCs did some of these many tasks very well, some did not do all of them and some did some of them badly. These many tasks were not all statutory responsibilities, such as helping patients and the public with information, advice and complaints – but they were expectations against which CHCs were judged.

Lack of guidance and relationship with management

While the lack of guidelines meant that CHCs were able to be innovative and creative, it also set them up to fail. According to the statutory regulations, NHS managers and CHCs were required to work together. The way the CHCs had been set up made friction inevitable. Most of the day-to-day tensions arose from the lack of clear guidance on the respective roles of both CHCs and the NHS. Managers were encouraged but not required to involve CHCs. They could exclude or include CHCs and encourage partnership or conflict. Family health services, a major part of healthcare, were excluded from the powers of CHCs.

The DHSS from the start failed to give guidance to CHCs and health authorities that might have reduced the tensions and conflicts that arose. In fact they made the situation harder by giving an expanded role to CHCs without clear boundaries between management and representation. CHC members were asked to obtain information about the services provided and sit in judgement on the adequacy of the NHS in their district. They were expected to understand statistical information needed to assess standards, investigate conditions or facilities and get involved in the planning process. Health authority members were also expected to assess standards, investigate conditions and get involved in the planning process.

Jack Hallas (1976) found that there was a crossover and entanglement between area health authorities and CHC members from an early stage as both set about making visits and getting to know the area. The potential friction in overlapping roles of health authorities and CHCs was exacerbated because many members of both CHCs and health authorities were appointed from the same local authority source. About two-fifths of CHC members appointed in 1974–75 had either been on a local authority health committee or a hospital management committee. Furthermore, local authority councillors were experienced in combining management and representative functions and some felt CHCs were irrelevant. They also resented that community health services had been transferred to the NHS in 1974. In spite of this, CHCs opposed linking of management and representation and felt that it was possible to separate them (Hallas, 1976).

The effectiveness of the CHC in influencing decisions depended greatly on the willingness of NHS managers to work with it. It did not take long for some NHS managers to learn how to manipulate CHCs. At one extreme a close relationship between the CHC and the district management team could undermine the independence and confidence of the CHC. In the West Midlands, one DHA involved the CHC in planning teams and joint activities from the start. The district administrator attended CHC meetings and dealt with questions as they arose. As a result the CHC never got to grips with its role since the answer was available at the first airing. The CHC began to meet five times a year instead of monthly and disbanded its working groups (Saunders, 1985). It is difficult to assess the effectiveness of CHCs or the impact they had in specific or general terms. Improvements might be carried out after recommendations by the CHC, but it is impossible to know whether the changes were made because the area health authority had decided to make those changes already, it was swayed by the evidence presented by the CHC or it wanted to avoid confrontation with the CHC.

Most disputes were not about local issues but attempts by CHCs to exert their rights: obtaining information and the right to be consulted. It was not clear how far CHCs had the right to information that was not readily available or where the district management team deemed it to be confidential or politically sensitive. A survey by the National Consumer Council and ACHCEW (1984) found wide variations in the information available to CHCs. Information that was offered as of a right by some district health authorities was treated as if it were classified by others. CHCs received little support from the DHSS in their battles to exert their right to information in order to carry out their functions. The DHSS was ambivalent about sharing information from Hospital Advisory Service (HAS) reports on long stay hospitals, though the HAS constantly complained that their recommendations were not followed up. These reports remained confidential and it was left to the discretion of area health authorities to share the recommendations of the report with CHCs. This apparent ambivalence of governments increased the variability among CHCs in their activities.

CHC members and theories of representation

CHCs had a 'uniquely eccentric' way of choosing members. It was very different to the consultative committees attached to the nationalised industries where members were picked by civil servants and lacked any sort of constituency in the community. The final arrangements for CHCs suggest an attempt to balance representation from the community with representation for special interests among NHS users. CHC members nominated by local authorities were broadly seen as representing the community in some undefined way. The third of CHC members chosen by voluntary organisations can be seen as an answer to the problem of ensuring representation of special interests but also recognised and promoted participation of the voluntary sector. This brought new people into the system. They may not have had so much experience in public representation (the strength of the local authority members) or experience in health service management (the contribution of the RHA nominees) but had extensive and wide experience of health and social services from a user perspective.

Underlying these arrangements for representation was a confusion of different theories of representation. Members may be selected as individuals, because they 'mirror' the social and economic structure of the community in terms of social class, education and demographic factors like age. As Klein and Lewis point out the usefulness of this approach is limited, since it treats representative bodies as though they were the permanent sample in an ongoing public opinion poll. The fact that people are prepared to put themselves forward for selection suggests they may be unrepresentative of the network from which they are recruited. Further, it is assumed that representation implies voicing the values, attitudes and experiences of those being represented which is not necessarily the case and which is why public opinion surveys use large samples. If the relevant community is seen to be users rather than the public at large there are also difficulties. Do you weight representation towards the intensity of use of services? In which case older people and children would need high levels of representation.

Alternatively, members can be selected because they represent groups in the community, patients or their agents. CHC appointments did not put value on the experiences of the individual, as happened later with patients' forums that replaced them, but on the groups that they represented, which enabled members to collect wider information from their networks and contacts within the community and among users. This, however, does not deal with the problem of how to get the views of people who are not part of normal networks and are not organised.

The accountability or legitimacy of members was never clear, however. Discussion focussed on the composition and representativeness of CHCs. Little attention was given to their accountability either to the public they served or for their use of public funds. Once appointed, members had collective loyalty to the NHS and were not expected to be individually accountable to the bodies that nominated them.

The verdict – a qualified success

The first few years can be seen as the golden age of CHCs. They were generally seen as a success story. In the first few years CHCs received favourable mentions in several government reports. They saw CHCs having an important role in implementing the polices they were promoting. The Court report on services for children, *Fit for the Future,* concluded: '*It is as yet early days to assess their effectiveness but we look to them to inject a fresh democratic note into health service planning. That they have a role to play is clear*' (DHSS, 1976b: 21.33). The report recommended that CHCs' rights be extended to primary care and that CHCs be able to request a visit by the Health Advisory Service, a national inspectorate for long stay hospitals. Dr David Owen, Minister of Health, in 1976 wrote of CHCs: '*the decision to establish community health councils will probably be looked back on by social historians as the most significant aspect of the whole of the NHS Reorganisation Act 1973. For the first time there exists a strong consumer body to both criticise and champion the NHS*' (Owen, 1976: 18). Ten years later, David Owen, now leader of the Social Democratic Party wrote another book on the NHS, that barely mentions CHCs (Owen, 1988). However, that was to come later.

CHCs, though not universally popular, were seen mostly as a positive force for bringing about change in the NHS and making it more responsive to its users. Through CHC membership voluntary organisations were for the first time recognised as a constituency in their own right. The King's Fund saw this as a crucial role and observed in evidence to the Royal Commission in 1979 '*that CHCs should aim to become a local focus for the encouragement of voluntary effort in support of the health services of the district*' (King's Fund, 1977: 35). In a survey in 1982 the overwhelming majority of district administrators were in favour of keeping CHCs and thought them a valuable institution, though many complained of the political activities of local authority councillors and the unwillingness of some CHCs to set priorities for the needs they uncovered (Bates, 1982).

The definitive verdict on the early years of CHCs was delivered by the Royal Commission on the NHS in its report in 1979. The Royal Commission report pointed to the uncertainty and confusion about the role of CHCs amongst CHCs, health authorities and other bodies. Conflicting opinions were expressed about how and when CHCs should be consulted and whether they should be given a formal part in decision-making. Many health authorities commented to the Commission on the positive part CHCs played in helping to develop health services in their districts. Criticisms of CHCs came from two sources: professionals and local government. Some professionals expressed hostility towards CHCs. They saw them as aggressive and destructive and felt that they prevented professionals from getting on with their job. Others felt that they lacked the power to be effective in representing user interests.

The Association of District Councils from a local authority perspective felt that CHCs would not be necessary if there was democratic management of the health service. However, in the absence of this the role of CHCs might be strengthened by giving them some powers of decision-making in relation to the assessment of priorities. Many CHCs submitted evidence that they felt they did not have the power or the resources to fulfil their functions effectively.

In summary, the Commission concluded: '*in our view CHCs have been an experiment which should be supported further..........They need to be involved at the formative stages of policy development. The Health Department should give them more specific advice on the role they are expected to play. If the structural changes recommended in chapter 20 are introduced it will be important that the close identification of CHCs with relatively small populations is retained*' (Royal Commission on the NHS, 1979: 11.11).

Rudolf Klein and Janet Lewis in 1976 carried out the first and, arguably, the last in-depth independent study of CHCs nationally. They concluded that the most important change that CHCs had brought might be in the culture of the NHS. If it had led to changes in the way in which administrators and professionals approached and perceived their task, the introduction of CHCs would have made a major difference to the NHS.

'*It is important to try to imagine what the reorganised NHS would be like if there were no CHCs. There would be no band of inquisitive men and women going round hospitals and other facilities asking the occasional awkward question or looking at the small change of patient comfort. There would be no one to argue the case of providing more information about what was happening in the NHS and pressing for a less introspective and more open style of decision-making. There would be no one to provide a platform for individuals or pressure groups – whether the rival fluoridation lobbies or the midwives seeking to exclude men from exercising their profession – who want to make their case heard or seek allies. There would be no institutionalised way of bringing official rhetoric about what is desirable face-to-face with the realities of what is happening local*' (Klein and Lewis, 1976: 156).

Conclusions

CHCs were set up as autonomous local bodies and this led to internal conflicts and limited their ability to develop as a movement and adapt to the changing world. While the lack of guidelines meant that CHCs were able to be innovative and creative, it also set them up to fail. They were set up with good intentions but little understanding of what consumer representation actually meant. They developed in different ways, taking different approaches. This led to innovation but also led to wide inconsistencies and variations, which undermined them as a national movement.

The early years were a good time to be involved in CHCs; there was general support from Government for what they were doing. There was often scepticism from the public who felt that 'the watchdog' had no teeth, and among professionals who felt that CHCs had too much power. However, there was scope to achieve a lot and given the wide remit and little guidance each CHC invented itself. NHS managers had little experience of dealing with the public or the voluntary sector and so it was possible to have a real influence on their thinking. However, it was clear by the end of the period that reform was needed. The strength of CHCs lay in their local autonomy but this also meant that there were increasing divisions between CHCs and how they saw their role. CHCs already felt that reform was needed to enable them to be effective.

However, this was not to be. The Conservative Government that came into office in 1979 had a different view. There was no place for a local consumer groups embedded in social rights of the post-war era.

Community Health Councils – The Decline 1979–1997

'CHCs were set up without a blueprint. They were given few rights, few resources and even fewer duties. Each has evolved its own personality. They were set up in an era when the fashionable ideology was community participation. They are in a metaphorical sense a relic of the last great campaign for community participation. Since then that they have been left to their own devices and ignored by the outside world.' Fedelma Winkler (1989: 8).

Overview

This chapter looks at how CHCs responded to the changes in the NHS after 1979 when they lost the support of Government which favoured individual consumer rights over social rights and collective approaches to engagement.

- From 1979 CHCs came under attack and there was a continual erosion of their role and rights.
- With the introduction of general management and the market, managers began to relate directly to their consumers leading to management-led consumerist approaches to participation.
- CHCs resisted attempts to make them relate to commissioners rather than providers and stop giving assistance to individuals.
- With an increasing workload and no additional resources, CHCs became increasingly divided and introverted as they debated reform and performance management.
- CHCs as independent autonomous bodies were not in a position to reform themselves.

Introduction

In 1979 CHCs had reason to feel optimistic about their future. The Royal Commission and other national bodies had recommended that they be strengthened and made more effective. They were hoping for more resources and reform. By 1981 some researchers had the impression that a large proportion of CHCs were just keeping their head above the water (Farrell and Adams, 1981). They were overwhelmed by the bureaucratic demands of paperwork from the NHS that they had to process. In those districts with many consultations on closures, CHCs were left with little time to do anything else.

However, the world had moved on even before the Royal Commission reported. In 1979 the Labour Government of James Callaghan was replaced by the Conservative Government of Margaret Thatcher. The next 18 years of Conservative Government were not friendly towards CHCs. During the 1970s the New Right had questioned the value of social rights – the basis of the welfare state. Campaigns against poor health standards or poverty had short-term successes, but they also provided evidence of the failures of the welfare state. This was a challenge to the tradition on which CHCs were based – collective approaches to participation that aimed to address inequalities. Policies now favoured consumer rights (see Chapter 6).

While the Government in the 1970s was generally supportive of CHCs, they had powerful enemies working behind the scenes. Doctors were locked in battle with the Labour Government about private practice and pay beds fighting for what they saw as their professional integrity. Patrick (later Lord) Jenkin, the Conservative spokesman for health, received regular hostile reports about CHCs from consultants and hospital managers during this period. Doubts about the continued existence of CHCs resulted from these regular discussions (Gerrard, 2006: 90). Roland Moyle, Labour Minister for Health from 1976, did not receive such reports which he attributed to the fact that government was in favour of CHCs and so there was little point in lobbying them (Gerrard, 2006: 215).

Patients First

In December 1979 the Government published its response to the Royal Commission in a consultative document, *Patients First*. This proposed to abolish one tier of administration, with district health authorities taking over the functions of both district management teams and area health authorities. The consultative paper questioned whether separate consumer representation in the form of CHCs would still be needed. Views were invited on whether CHCs should be retained (DHSS, 1979).

There was wide opposition to the abolition of CHCs from the public and all political parties and the future of CHCs generated more responses than any other issue in *Patients First*. Members of the public wrote to record their support for CHCs, in some cases relating the personal stories of how their CHC had helped them. Of the nearly 5000 comments relating to CHCs, over half were from members of the public. The reasons that were given for the retention of CHCs included the belief that representation and management were separate and required a different perspective and different skills. CHCs were also supported because they were champions of Cinderella services – a particularly important role in districts where consultants in acute services were very powerful. Members of the public felt their views had more weight when expressed though the CHC.

The only substantial opposition came from the medical profession and NHS managers (DHSS, 1980). Those who wanted to abolish CHCs characterised them as disruptive and unnecessary pressure groups, often politically motivated, with no clear purpose or effect. Some suggested how CHCs might be modified if they were retained. Suggestions included a review of the terms of reference of CHCs; reducing their membership; increasing voluntary organisation representation at the expense of local authority members; reducing CHCs' power generally and specifically in respect of their ability to intervene in closures; increasing their powers and resources and mounting a national publicity campaign.

By February 1980 Patrick Jenkin told a special meeting of CHCs convened by ACHCEW that the case for keeping CHCs in place was 'formidable'. On 23 July 1980 the Secretary of State announced that CHCs were to be retained with a review to follow in three years (DHSS, 1980).

The aftermath

CHCs had received outstanding support, but their problems were only beginning. After *Patients First* there was a continual erosion of the status and powers of CHCs. It seems that CHCs had one important enemy, the Minister of Health, Dr Gerald Vaughan, who had been a consultant child psychiatrist, and opposed the setting up of the national association in 1977.[1] He had wanted to get rid of CHCs. Thwarted by the strength of the support for CHCs, he tackled the issue from another angle, in particular attacking CHC activities at national level.

A consultation document, *The Role of Community Health Councils,* was published in 1981. CHCs were told that there would be no more resources and they would have fewer members. It proposed limiting CHC complaints work. It was also proposed that CHCs should cease to be independent of the authorities they were supposed to scrutinise and that the new district health authorities should become their establishing body, including appointing members (DHSS, 1981). This was a step too far and in the subsequent guidance RHAs remained the establishing body and CHCs kept their independence.

The only change was the reduction of members to 18 to 25 members, compared to 22 to 33 members previously. Ministers felt that smaller CHCs would be more effective and that they did not think it was right for CHCs to have a membership larger than that of the district health authority to which they related. This illustrates the continuing misunderstandings about the role of members of CHCs and health authorities. Health authority members were appointed to manage the service, CHCs to represent the community. The number of members necessary for an efficient management body is not related to the number needed for an effective representative body. Many CHCs felt that the reduction in membership decreased the direct representation of different sections of the community on the CHC as well as the number of volunteers available to carry out CHC business.

CHCs and national activities

The government could not get rid of CHCs because they had so many allies at local level, but ACHCEW was an easier target. CHCs were told that ministers saw them as local bodies without a voice in the NHS at national level. If CHCs were to be local bodies only, they did not need a national association, particularly one that saw its role as questioning government policies, which was something ACHCEW was increasingly confident in doing. For example, in 1981 the Association of CHCs for England and Wales held a special conference devoted to the Black Report on health inequalities whose recommendations had been rejected by the Government and adopted a resolution that deplored its response.

The first target was *CHC News*, a popular and high profile monthly newsletter. The Government withdrew its funding. *CHC News* continued paid for by subscription for a short time but published its final edition in March 1984. Mike Gerrard, the Director of ACHCEW at the time, observes: '*I am certain that, finding CHCs themselves too determined and resilient to put down easily, and too popular in some quite unexpected quarters to make their demise politically acceptable, the government decided to go for their weak spot, and shut off the funding for their information service. In this way, ministers were able to terminate a commitment made by their predecessors, silence a persistent critic, and reduce the operational capacity of CHCs by removing their information and communication mechanism at a stroke*' (Gerrard, 2006: 118).

The next target was the national association. ACHCEW had a troubled beginning with less than full support from CHCs and it was easy to cause further divisions among CHCs. In 1981 the DHSS announced that funding would be withdrawn from ACHCEW over two years. This resulted in a financial crisis in 1983, when ACHCEW nearly closed down. In the end the DHSS provided deficit funding for the following two years. In 1984 at a special general meeting CHCs agreed to continue to support ACHCEW and to fund it from subscriptions based on budget allocations. In 1983, 205 out of 217 CHCs were in membership, this declined to 175 in 1985.

Respite came in 1983 when the new Minister, Kenneth Clarke, assured an ACHCEW AGM that that their future was not at risk. In 1985 the DHSS restored the grant to ACHCEW. Thereafter CHCs were ignored, not worth the effort required to abolish them. There was disappointment among CHCs that the Government did not undertake the promised review of CHCs in 1983. CHCs were confident that a review would have endorsed them and provided additional resources. ACHCEW, under a new director, Tony Smythe, started to recover some confidence after the difficult years following the loss of government funding. ACHCEW commissioned a report to look at how CHCs had developed, what they had achieved and how CHCs might adapt to the changes in the NHS (Hogg, 1986). The report encouraged CHCs to address issues like standards and quality in their own performance. It made recommendations about how CHCs could provide a framework for public participation in the future and what changes would be required, including clarification of rights and duties, codes of practice, budgets and staffing that reflected the work, and a review of the way that members were selected. The report was overwhelmingly approved at ACHCEW's annual general meeting in July 1986. The report was followed up by a report on examples of good practice in CHCs (Hogg, 1987). This was the first attempt to set standards. It looked like CHCs were waking up to the need to change and adapt to the new environment in which they were working. However, CHCs remained essentially local autonomous bodies and were not prepared to give up their freedom of action at the cost of standardisation. So these initiatives like many others in the 1990s were not followed through by action. ACHCEW could encourage good practice, but there were no carrots or sticks that it could use with CHCs.

In the long-term closure of *CHC News* and undermining the national association were destructive for CHCs, encouraging divisions and making it harder for the movement to work together to reform itself. There were concerns about the attempt to stifle CHCs. Farrell and Adams (1981) noted that national policies aimed to set standards that were responsive to local needs and that it seemed wasteful and undemocratic not to allow CHCs, which represent the public interest, to have some influence on national policies.

It is not perhaps surprising that the new Conservative Government had fallen out of love with CHCs. While there was consensus about the general direction of the NHS and government policies, CHCs were useful to them. When the consensus ended, CHCs were no longer useful in implementing government policies, and, in fact, became an obstacle to them. CHCs had added additional stresses into the health system. They had strong local loyalty and were involved in battles, not just to redistribute resources between services within their districts, but to increase the amount of resources for their districts. They had opened up the NHS to much more scrutiny and politicised issues. They were equally willing to criticise government as their local NHS management and many were adept at using the media to publicise their causes at national and local level.

General management

The next change to sideline CHCs was the introduction of general management in 1983. Roy Griffiths, Chairman of Sainsbury's, was commissioned to inquire into how the management of the NHS might be improved (DHSS, 1983). Up till then the NHS had been 'administered' rather than 'managed'. General management meant that one identified manager, rather than a management team, took responsibility. There was a belief that management was a transferable skill – as long as you understood management you did not need to understand the NHS, your locality or the politics of health. The Griffiths report saw the end of consensus management. General management aimed to make top-down reform possible and enable managers to intervene in clinical management.

Roy Griffiths criticised the NHS for its lack of attention to its consumers and encouraged them to relate directly to their consumers and undertake consumer surveys. He reported that he had been impressed with the grass roots work of some CHCs (DHSS, 1983). CHCs lost the monopoly that they had enjoyed in the 1970s. There were increasingly other ways that managers could relate to 'consumers' both through their own activities and voluntary organisations. This led to a management-led consumerist approach, which tended to look at the hotel aspects of services, such as food and cleanliness, rather than the effectiveness of services (Klein, 2001). Griffiths was deeply concerned about the impact on NHS consultation procedures on the efficiency of the service. *'By any business standards the process of consultation is so labyrinthine and the right to veto so considerable, that the result in many cases is institutionalised stagnation'* (DHSS, 1983: 12). In 1985 regulations removed the automatic right to be consulted from CHCs. This is discussed Chapter 5.

The introduction of general management changed the relationship of CHCs with management. Much of a CHC's influence depended on the willingness of managers to listen and to negotiate. However, the new general managers were on short-term contracts; they did not necessarily have a background in the NHS or a long-term commitment to the locality. They were going places and did not have the time or interest to build relationships and trust with the CHC. No longer protected by the support of government, attitudes to CHCs among NHS managers changed during the 1980s. In a survey in 1985, 71 percent of district general managers considered that CHCs had played a useful role in making the NHS more aware of patients needs (Saunders, 1985). However, many were not convinced that CHCs were still needed. They were asked if the CHC did not exist would they establish one in their district and 36 percent said yes but nearly half said no. With managers less willing to listen and to be influenced, CHCs became increasingly marginalised.

During this time CHCs, who had already been complaining that lack of resources limited their effectiveness, became even more stretched as their workload increased. In 1985 CHCs' remit had been extended to give them the same rights towards family practitioner committees as they had with district health authorities (DHSS, 1985). Patients' expectations were rising, and they were looking to the CHCs for information and advice. Most CHCs continued to provide information and advice to the public and assist complainants. As a result a sense of frustration built up and continued to do so through the 1980s and 1990s. Pickard (1997) concluded that CHCs workload had increased while funding was unchanged and this had diluted CHCs' capacity to provide an effective service. The very existence of CHCs had unquestionably hinged in the last few years on the willingness of CHC chief officers in particular to work many unpaid hours overtime each week.

Purchasers and providers

NHS reforms had not delivered either efficiency or votes for the Government. The same problems remained. Providers still shaped the debate and there were constant horror stories in the media with clinicians 'shroud waving' to try to get more resources for their services. Margaret Thatcher had changed the face of Britain during the 1980s, taking on the trade unions, privatising the nationalised industries and selling off public housing. Now it was time to take on the NHS and she announced the NHS Review in 1988.

The white paper, *Working for Patients,* and the NHS and Community Care Act 1990 set up the conditions for a healthcare market and marked the end of any attempt at consensus, see Box 4.1 (DH, 1989). Proposals were based on a view of society that believed people should be free to buy better or more services, if they could afford it. Consumers are meant to be the driver for change who can exert their right to choose or to refuse a service. As a result, it was hoped, popular services would prosper and less popular ones decline. This was in direct contrast with the values of the NHS that for 40 years had emphasised the importance of collective responsibility and equal access to medical care regardless of financial, social or cultural constraints (Townsend and Davidson, 1988).

Working for Patients, only briefly mentioned CHCs. They would continue but the Government wanted them to focus on working with commissioners, rather than monitoring providers. The rights they had to be an observer at board meetings, to information, to make visits and be consulted remained with the health authorities and were not extended to NHS trusts or fundholding GPs. It was suggested once again that CHCs should give up working with individual complainants. CHCs' traditional role of being consulted on substantial service changes was whittled away. In 1985 regulations removed the automatic right to be consulted from CHCs. This is discussed Chapter 5.

Box 4.1   The NHS and Community Care Act 1990

District health authorities became **purchasers** responsible for assessing the health needs of their population and purchasing services on their behalf. They lost their elected local authority representatives and had fewer members, with chairman and non-executive directors appointed by the Secretary of State rather than regional health authorities.

NHS hospitals were able to become **self-governing trusts**, independent of health authorities and accountable to the Secretary of State.

Family practitioner committees became **family health service authorities** with responsibility for managing and planning primary care rather than just administering services.

Larger GP practices were encouraged to manage their own budgets as **fundholders** and contract a specific range of services for their patients.

The purchaser/provider split was introduced into local authority social services and they were required to publish **community care plans**, where possible, jointly with the health authority.

Source: The NHS and Community Care Act 1990

It was a harder environment for CHCs in which to operate. With choice, the 'voice' traditionally provided by CHCs was less important. Consumers can use their right to exit and choose an alternative service or complain. With the proliferation of providers the NHS became more complex; with a focus on contracts and their specifications. It was not clear that CHC members would have the skills and expertise to monitor contracts. It did, though, recognise the potential conflicts between health authorities who were responsible for planning (or commissioning as it was now called) and those providing services. The implicit assumption behind the creation of CHCs was that the interests of the consumer were different from those of the providers of healthcare. The purchaser/provider split recognised this.

CHCs and commissioning

The Department of Health saw the future of CHCs to be less confrontational, working with health authorities in identifying unmet needs and acting as an advocate for local communities. Government encouraged NHS bodies to directly seek the views of people and build up relationships with the voluntary sector. The publication of guidance, *Local Voices,* from the NHS Management Executive seemed a major breakthrough for the voluntary sector (NHSME, 1992). With increased direct involvement of voluntary groups, it was harder for CHCs to maintain their legitimacy as representatives of the public interest. It better fitted with the role of the CHC as a facilitator of local voices, which many CHCs had adopted. As user-led and advocacy groups became more established, they did not feel they needed a mediating agency, such as the CHC.

There were opportunities for CHCs as the established experts on involving users and in finding out the views of consumers. For health authorities CHCs' local knowledge could be valuable as well as their ability to facilitate joint working with the voluntary sector. However, the new health authorities covered large areas, sometimes whole counties such as Devon, so the usefulness of CHCs depended on their willingness to work together. This was something that CHCs, noted for their insularity and individuality, were not good at doing. Sometimes differences between local communities and their health concerns were sufficiently great to render attempts to work together unsuccessful, though it often seemed to come down to personalities (Pickard, 1997).

At this time there were debates about how healthcare might be rationed and a hope that CHCs might take on a role in helping commissioners choose priorities. This was an area that most CHCs were reluctant to get involved in. Some were suspicious that this was a means to get them to legitimise cuts in services (ACHCEW, 1993).

From 1996 the Department of Health began to promote the idea of patient partnerships, indicating that it wanted the NHS to engage with the public and patients directly, bypassing CHCs. The patient partnership strategy aimed to promote service users' involvement in their own care and encourage informed choice as well as developing health services overall to make the

NHS more responsive to the needs and preferences of users; and to support effective involvement of users (NHSE, 1996). The strategy saw a role for CHCs in monitoring elements of the patient partnership strategy.

CHCs and NHS trusts

Traditionally CHCs had worked closely with providers in monitoring services: visiting, attending meetings and carrying out surveys. CHCs and ACHCEW resisted the proposed change to their traditional ways of working. CHCs wanted to retain their dual focus and role with providers (ACHCEW, 1989). They did not want to give up any activities, wanted to take on new activities and the resources to do them.

Initially providers reported little change in the relationship with CHCs, but relations were becoming confused. The options available to CHCs were to either work with providers and help them with their consumer activities, or retain their vision and be more proactive and confrontational (Moon and

---

Box 4.2   Types of CHCs

Collaborative CHCs

DHA partners – CHCs that worked closely with the DHA and were involved in decision-making. They were also more likely than other types to 'sell' DHA/FHSA plans to the public. Though concerned with individual consumer complaints, they did not always take the side of the consumer.

Patients' friend – CHCs that worked for individual consumers rather than general consumer rights and were particularly concerned with individual complaints. They were not closely involved with the DHA and were excluded from decision-making. They saw themselves on the side of the consumer acting as an arbiter between consumers and the DHA.

Consumer advocate – CHCs that were actively working to consumers' rights but using existing structures. They appreciated the importance of working with the Health Authority and were involved to a certain extent in decision-making. They were more likely than any other of the types to see themselves as being on the consumer's side.

Independent CHCs

Independent challengers – CHCs that saw themselves on the side of the consumer working for collective consumer rights, challenging the government but not working closely with the DHA and had excluded themselves from decision-making.

Independent arbiters – CHCs that saw their primary role as an independent arbiter between consumers and the DHA and not taking the side of either. They did not see their primary role as being one of pursuing consumer complaints nor do they feel they were necessarily on the side of the consumer.

Source: Buckland et al., 1995.

Lupton, 1995). If CHCs became directly involved in consumer activities in acute services, they might lose their vision of popular democracy, and take on the role of an independent evaluator. The differences in how CHCs saw their role and their capacity to adapt to the changing world were illustrated in research by Buckland and colleagues (1995). They identified five types of CHCs based on a national attitude survey of CHC chief officers (see Box 4.2). Broadly some CHCs aimed to collaborate with the NHS, while others feared this would compromise their independence. The study concluded that collaborative CHCs (patients' friend, health authority partner and consumer advocates) were more highly valued and regarded by the health authority and trust managers. The two independent types had not really understood the changes in the NHS or adapted to new ways of working. The study also found that staffing of collaborative CHCs was greater than in other CHCs – each had three or more staff, though not necessarily full time.

The case for CHC reform

When the NHS Review was published in 1989, shock waves reverberated. It was clear that this was a different vision for the NHS and not merely tinkering with the administrative arrangements. NHS managers, academics and professionals, who distrusted the changes, wanted a strong patients' voice to speak out and campaign against the proposals – which were seen as the beginning of marketisation. CHCs were the obvious vehicle to do this and, for a short time, there was an interest in developing a stronger role for CHCs among managers. At a conference organised for London CHCs, Maureen Dixon, Institute of Health Service Management, outlined how the Institute had come to the conclusion that there is a need for a counter-bureaucracy in the NHS (Dixon, 1989). She pointed out that with the internal market there was a potential for fragmentation of services and that a powerful pressure group for patients at national and regional levels to support and co-ordinate the local consumer bodies could be an important force to prevent this. David Hunter, then Director of the Nuffield Institute of Health Services Studies, pointed out that if CHCs were to take advantage of opportunities they would need to be clearer about their values and the model of consumerism they upheld (Hunter, 1989). Some people involved in CHCs felt that there were opportunities for CHCs to rethink their purpose and organisation. At a conference for CHCs in 1989 the author warned, in retrospect prophetically: 'CHCs have been left far behind and we have a lot of catching up to do. CHCs can provide the framework for consumer representation, but not the way they are now. If CHCs go for radical rather than sticking plaster solutions, they risk some vicious battles, which may split CHCs into factions. The alternative is that CHCs will continue to die a slow death. The experiences of CHCs and the basic framework of community involvement will be lost – to the great detriment of health service users' (Hogg, 1989: 9).

These were challenges that CHCs and ACHCEW did not take up. ACHCEW fought during the 1990s to maintain the status quo, retaining a role for CHCs with both purchasers and providers. CHCs were demanding more resources and marginal change but not facing up to the real situation. While the Government encouraged the NHS to by-pass CHCs and go out and meet their communities and encouraged the voluntary sector to become service providers and compete in the market, CHCs became increasingly introverted and absorbed with internal debates about what they wanted and how the Government might be persuaded to give it to them. Often the only agree-ment seemed to be the need for more resources to reflect their increasing workload.

CHCs were autonomous bodies that valued their freedom of action and could not change by themselves; they needed external and legislative changes. ACHCEW could identify good practice and propose standards for CHCs per-formance, but could not impose anything on individual CHCs. Perhaps the hope for CHCs lay in their willingness to work together to suggest acceptable plans for reform. But that was not the way of CHCs.

There were attempts to think about radical reform and several reports were published. The Institute of Health Service Management and ACHCEW commissioned a paper on future options, *Back From the Margins*. This looked at different models for community participation and favoured the re-establishment of CHCs based on a community development model, with the role of engaging and facilitating groups and individuals to take part, rather than directly representing the public (Hogg, 1996). Chris Dabbs, Chief Officer at Salford CHC, in his report *At the Crossroads* (1998), advocated relinquishing the complaints service and honing down CHCs' role to one of four options: independent monitoring and scrutiny of service provision and commissioning; facilitation and co-ordination of lay involvement and participation in service provision and commissioning; independent moni-toring and scrutiny of public health improvement; or facilitation and coordination of lay involvement and participation in public health/health improvement.

Performance standards – the search for the Holy Grail

The continuing need for CHCs was not widely questioned, but they were criticised for their variability. It was the accepted wisdom that CHCs were inconsistent and variable, though there was no evidence for what this actually meant in terms of quality of service. Managers, the main source of informa-tion on variability, were not necessarily objective. Cooper et al. (1996) pointed out that some CHCs were able to fulfil part or all of their respons-ibilities with a degree of success, but much depended on the personality and skills of individuals concerned. Variations may well be a benefit, reflecting local priorities but this could increase the sense that they were inconsistent and variable. The more important issue was how the CHC set and reviewed its objectives and the framework for accountability.

The key to the survival of CHCs in the 1990s seemed to be to refute the allegations of variability and inconsistency. Performance management and standards were being introduced into the NHS, but there were no arrangements to set performance standards for CHCs, staff or members. Regional health authorities, as the establishing bodies, had responsibility to ensure that services they funded met user's needs and fulfilled their statutory duties. However, there were no agreed standards against which CHC performance could be measured. It was felt that it would be better for CHCs to set their own standards and priorities, otherwise their independence would be undermined as regional health authorities were part of the system that CHCs were set up to monitor. An executive letter from the Department of Health in 1994 stated that CHCs were expected to produce an annual plan and that regions should discuss with CHCs their progress and the use they made of their resources (DH, 1994a).

Defining an effective CHC and developing performance standards dominated the 1990s – the search for the Holy Grail in Mike Gerrard's phrase. CHCs became increasingly inward looking searching for performance standards, which might help them survive, and in balancing the increased workload and expectations without additional resources. The problem was that there was no clear understanding of what CHCs were to do. Because of the lack of guidance, CHCs could be good or bad in so many different ways. Among CHCs there was also debates about whether services to the individual such as complaints advocacy, information and advice, were appropriate to combine with the wider of functions of representing the views of the public in service planning.

While ACHCEW accepted that there had to be a process for reviewing activities, it felt that the policies and priorities of the individual CHC must remain with them (Harris, 1995). There was widespread support within CHCs for greater consistency and an adoption of core standards. ACHCEW produced some performance standards for CHCs (Hogg, 1994a). At the AGM in 1994, the performance standards were accepted and recommended to all CHCs. However, there were no mechanisms to monitor their implementation or processes of review. Many CHCs developed a process of peer review in order to set the work plan with targets that they could then review a year later (Arnold et al., 1992). This helped some CHCs to change and focus more on community development activity. The number of projects increased rapidly between 1996 and 1998, inspired by the growing confidence the self review process conferred (Gerrard, 2006). However, many CHCs failed to engage with these processes (Pickard, 1997).

Concerns with performance standards were also tied up with accountability. It was never clear to whom CHCs were accountable and the relationship they had to their community or appointing organisations. In a survey of CHC members 95 percent of respondents saw accountability to local people to be a high priority, but few recognised the need to extend this beyond the annual report and AGM. A survey and report carried out by CHC chief officers observed that CHCs might not yet be ready to accept the challenge of demonstrating their accountability to local communities (Arnold et al., 1995b).

Insight

Regional health authorities were abolished in 1995 and replaced by regional offices of the NHS Executive. Regional offices, whose main responsibility was the performance management of the NHS, became the establishing bodies for CHCs but were to provide a 'light touch' management in providing support to CHCs and the monitoring of their performance (DH, 1995). CHCs became increasingly concerned about interference from the regional offices, that would in the long-term undermine their independence.[2]

The variations between CHCs had been exacerbated from the start by different ways that regional health authorities managed and funded CHCs. These differences now came into stark focus and the Department of Health wanted to address the variations in regional policies towards CHCs – in accommodation, staffing, scope and scale of CHCs work and their performance. To tackle this issue the Department of Health commissioned Insight Consulting, its management consultancy arm, to review the resourcing and performance management of CHCs. The purpose of the review was to identify an equitable and consistent method for allocating resources across CHCs in England. However, in order to do this they needed to understand what a CHC was and what it should do. This in effect meant a review of their role and functions.

The Insight Report was the long awaited review that had been first promised in 1980. The report was sympathetic to CHCs. Its first conclusion was that CHCs had delivered an excellent service and proven to be adept at understanding public health interests in their broadest sense and bringing this to the attention of those who can improve those services. In other cases, it noted, they had developed and provided services themselves where they have identified gaps in local provision. It supported CHC's independent position which it saw as central to their achievements so far (Insight Consulting, 1996).

Insight Consulting (1996) based their report on a 'notional' CHC. It noted that CHCs were engaged in four core activities: consultation with health authorities and the public; monitoring local health services; providing information and advice; and a complaints handling service. Insight had proposed that CHCs should focus on consultation and a targeted investigation function working jointly with health authorities in commissioning and planning services. It felt that the traditional monitoring role, exemplified in visiting hospitals, was no longer an effective use of resources. Instead of monitoring services, CHCs should look at community needs and interests in specific areas of healthcare. Their work should be based on projects rather than a general overview of services. The report concluded that, from its fieldwork, the majority of CHCs were already taking this approach. Insight recommended an approach used in Gwent and Clwyd in Wales where there was a centralised CHC administration with local area committees reporting to the main CHC.

They recommended that the role of helping individuals and scrutiny should be separated (see Box 4.3). CHCs should stop providing information and advice and support to complainants, which was a non-statutory function.

> ### Box 4.3 Combining representation and complaints
>
> The combined CHC role for community representation and helping individuals had been accepted in the early days. However, Rudolf Klein and Janet Lewis had questioned whether this was appropriate as early as 1976. They found that CHCs were dispensing comfort, reassurance and advice to worried or lonely people, whose complaints were less a criticism of the NHS than a plea for someone to take an interest in their problems. They concluded that CHCs might end up playing a role for which they were never designed. They saw it as an expensive way of advertising the existence of CHCs to the public when there were other under financed advice-giving agencies.
>
> With abolition, many CHCs felt that important information about patients' experiences would be lost to the new patients' forums if complaints advocacy was undertaken by a separate agency. In the Parliamentary debates in 2002, the Government conceded that forums covering primary care trusts would provide ICAS – either through their own staff or by commissioning someone else to do this.
>
> This was never implemented and commissioning ICAS remained with the Department of Health and was contracted to voluntary organisations. It had been planned to pass over the responsibility for ICAS to the Commission for Patient and Public Involvement in Health (CPPIH), but the Department of Health retained resources and the overall management for ICAS. There were already pilots where other organisations were providing ICAS and they felt they were working well. There was concern about the idea of these being run and managed by 300 PCT forums and the capacity of CPPIH to manage them.

As the workload grew, complaints overwhelmed some CHC staff (Hogg, 1995). Most CHCs gave priority to people who asked for help but this affected the other activities they could take on since it was impossible to predict the number of complaints that would be received or the amount of work each would entail. Insight Management Consultants (1996) noted there was a very wide variation among CHCs in their commitment to working with complainants – from 30 complaints in one year in one CHC to 642 in another. However, they found that 42 percent of staff time was taken up in assisting individuals. Maintaining public access to an information and advice service could be difficult since CHC staff had to be out of the office from time to time and for safety reasons staff should not be alone in an office that is open to public callers. The consultants concluded that helping individuals was time consuming and might not be a cost effective use of time. They noted that the low numbers of callers with an average of less than two people a day did not merit the resources required to make the service available. In particular, they attacked the use of high street premises, which 18 percent of CHCs had and had been supported by the Royal Commission in 1979. They concluded that this role would no longer be required because of improvement in the NHS complaints procedure and the development of customer service functions in hospitals.

Having decided what CHCs should do in the future, the report went on to look at performance management. It recommended the adoption of explicit qualitative and quantitive performance measures, building on arrangements that were already in place for some CHCs with internal and peer review. The report then considered the basis for CHC funding, pointing out that there was no logical basis for allocations which varied from between 21.7p to 62p per head of population. Insight recommended that allocations should shift towards reflecting the regional allocations for health and community health services funding.

There was disappointment that Insight Consulting had ducked their main task which was to develop a resourcing formula. They recommended that CHCs should be funded according to population with no account taken of what CHCs did or the quality of their work. Perhaps the final disappointment was that it seemed at the time, and now even more, a retrospective report. It looked at what CHCs were in 1995 but did not look at what changes there might be or the strains that CHCs were experiencing. However, more drastic measures were needed. There was an entrenched diversity and attachment to locality and independence that CHCs from different viewpoints and different political stances shared.

The Insight report did not lead to a constructive debate among CHCs.[3] If Insight had recommended ways of using resources to reinforce good practice, CHCs might have engaged in a debate. ACHCEW's response was a paper with its own recommendations, mainly about the notional CHC (ACHCEW, 1997). It served as a '*de facto rejection of Insight, diffusing the argument and shifting official thinking away from the recommendations the consultants had made*' (Gerrard, 2006: 149). Another opportunity, perhaps the best opportunity, to reform CHCs was lost. At the 1998 AGM, CHCs accepted core policy priorities, as recommended by Insight. However, these core policies were ambitious and presupposed additional resources. The core principles continued to focus on issues outside the CHC's statutory remit, such as working with primary care groups and assisting complainants and promoting good health. CHCs were not willing to give up activities they were doing and they felt were valuable.

The search for a performance framework still continued. Sterile and circular arguments ground on about performance standards between ACHCEW and the Department of Health. In the South West region in the absence of national progress, a group of CHC chief officers developed a framework to evaluate the performance of local CHCs, including feedback from those working with and alongside the CHC (Rolfe et al., 1998). They recommended that the CHC might be a local partner for the Commission for Health Improvement (CHI) that was being set up as an inspectorate for the NHS. Discussions continued but ACHCEW had no mandate from members. The performance evaluation framework had not been agreed by October 1998, by which time the Director, Toby Harris had left to become Lord Harris of Haringey.

So nothing happened. Department of Health issued guidance that made some piecemeal attempts at reform, mainly in relation to members. There had been increasing problems in recruiting members in the 1990s and many existing members did not give the time required. The Government attempted to tackle the problem of uncommitted members by reducing the period of non-attendance at meetings from six months to four after which members could be dismissed. It also removed the age bar on members over 70 and urged the establishing bodies to aim for balance of representation in race, age, gender and geographical localities.

National representation

Toby Harris had replaced Tony Smythe as Director of ACHCEW in 1986. He saw his task as to get CHCs into a state where they could fight the next attempt to abolish them. However this was an uphill task. ACHCEW did not become the patients' voice envisaged by the DHSS in 1975. Some of the problems of ACHCEW up to 1983 were internal, caused by resource difficulties and disputes about the purpose of *CHC News* and the Association. However, the basic cause goes back again to the nature of CHCs and the way ACHCEW had been set up.

Firstly, CHCs did not have a clear overall philosophy, compared to voluntary organisations. People become involved with voluntary organisations because of their personal commitment to the aims of the organisation. The underlying philosophy of CHCs was a belief in the NHS and a role for its users. However, the NHS represents many diverse and conflicting interests and ways of providing healthcare. There were different views of their role between Conservative or Labour dominated CHCs, between the North and South. There were tensions between CHCs in cities and rural areas. The antagonism between London and other CHCs had developed at the very beginning. It was partly a difference in culture, but exacerbated by attempts to equalise NHS spending between geographical regions. London with its rich teaching hospitals was a loser under the RAWP formula and faced cuts.

Secondly, ACHCEW's funding depended on CHCs remaining in membership. Members paid their subscriptions and if ACHCEW tried anything they did not like they pulled out of membership or attempted to undermine the Director and Chair. ACHCEW had been set up without the wholehearted support from CHCs, who were suspicious that they would lose their independence and be associated with views they did not share. ACHCEW had to tread carefully to keep a consensus among CHCs with opposing views. It was impossible to address the variability of CHCs.

Thirdly, even before ACHCEW was set up there had been conflicts between members and staff about their respective roles and who 'owned' the CHC. Mostly staff and members worked well at local level, but there were always tensions within ACHCEW. Toby Harris was the first director to formally address the AGM. Before that Tony Smythe had been allowed to speak to a motion on mental health in prisons, an area where he was knowledgeable, but this had caused consternation. On the standing committee when ACHCEW was set up there were 26 members and four staff observers and members. This had changed from a four to one ratio to a two to one when the size of the management committee was reduced.

Fourthly, CHCs had a strong local loyalty and gave priority to their own districts. They often saw work undertaken at national and regional level as detracting from what members and staff could achieve locally. The ratio of paid staff to voluntary members also restricted the activities in which a CHC could be involved.

Fifthly, the lack of strong regional structures made it difficult for ACHCEW to build up and maintains strong links with its membership. It tended to relate to members individually, which reduced the possibilities of learning and sharing from each other's experiences.

Meanwhile elsewhere

Meanwhile, there were changes in other parts of the UK. In Northern Ireland the district committees, set up in 1974, had been replaced in 1991 by local health and social services councils attached to each of the four health boards, based very much on the model of CHCs. During the 1990s the Welsh CHCs, who were considered to be among the most resistant to change, became more separatist and stopped coming to the annual conference. The Welsh chief officers singing rugby songs in the bar had been a feature of the ACHCEW AGM for many years and stopped as fewer Welsh CHCs attended.

In Scotland there had been a major reorganisation in 1993 when the number of local health councils (LHCs) was reduced to 16 from 34 to match the new health boards. This meant that the councils had more staff and became more strategic. Though they still had a geographic perspective, they lost the local focus that they had had. In 1996 the Scottish Office commissioned Jim Eckford, a former Board Chief Executive, to undertake a review of LHCs, including their role, the appointment of members and forward planning.[4] By and large it gave LHCs a good report and said they were serving the public interest well but needed to be more consistent in their operation. A particular concern was the Association of Local Health Councils where membership was voluntary. In England ACHCEW could afford to lose a few CHCs in membership, but with a membership of only 16, every member mattered.

Variability in performance and in interpretation of the role were issues in all three countries. There were also issues about representation. On the whole most members of LHCs and health and social services councils preferred to represent their own views and did not see their role as going out to the community and council membership was seen to be less diverse than in England.

Conclusions

CHCs were set up at a different time with different values and new challenges came with the introduction of general management and the internal market with the focus on the patient as consumer, rather than collective approaches. The introduction of the internal market presented a challenge that CHCs were not equipped to meet without external help. During the 1990s Government pursued different means of involving the public and encouraging patients to act as consumers and CHCs remained struggling, increasingly marginalised and introspective.

Amazingly in the face of all these changes, CHCs survived the Thatcher years, though not unscathed. Reforms reduced their powers and membership and curtailed the activities of the national association, ACHCEW. Tensions were evident with the NHS as CHCs found themselves increasingly marginalised. By the end of the 1990s it was clear to many people, inside the CHC movement, that CHCs days were numbered. CHCs had become a side show, though the good work many did was still widely recognised.

The general verdict seems to have been that CHCs had not lived up to their potential. Historian Charles Webster (2002: 160) concluded '*CHCs survived although sometimes troublesome they were not particularly influential.*' CHCs now barely receive a mention in books on health policy. But these verdicts underestimate the impact that the existence of a local informed group had on the culture of the NHS, in particularly in holding the government to account and promoting the interests of 'Cinderella' services and of vulnerable groups who received and still receive poorer services. Many innovations to the NHS were pioneered by CHCs – advocacy, surveys, community development projects, patient support groups. Many MPs, members of the House of Lords and NHS board members gained experience and understanding about healthcare as CHC members, which was often an early stage in a political career. What was lost with CHCs was a local and national focus for informed and deliberative debate about health policy and practice, which leads to more robust and transparent decision-making.

Tackling the
Democratic Deficit

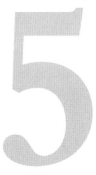

'Everyone is for participation … it can't be bad. But who is able to say what it is?' Sherri Arnstein, 1969: 216.

Overview

This chapter traces the way that governments have attempted to overcome the democratic deficit in the NHS.

- CHCs were set up as independent bodies mediating between the NHS and the public with rights to be consulted.
- From the 1980s NHS managers sought to consult their communities directly using a range of different techniques.
- In 2001 Overview and Scrutiny Committees (OSCs) took over some of the functions of CHCs and all NHS bodies were given a duty to consult the public.
- Mainstreaming participation has led to increased management control over the processes of participation and a focus on consumerist rather than democratic approaches.

Introduction

The decision to set up the National Health Service (NHS) as a separate organisation in 1948 directly responsible to the Secretary of State, left the NHS with a democratic deficit. Local government with elected councillors can claim to be representative in a way that health authority members could not. One of the main themes running through the Parliamentary debates on the reorganisation was the often reiterated belief that the presence of local authority members – whether on CHCs or health authorities – would in itself inject an element of democracy into the system (Klein and Lewis, 1976). The establishment of CHCs in 1974 was the first attempt to address the democratic deficit in the NHS. Among the many hopes for CHCs was that they would help to bridge the gap between the NHS and local authorities.

Half the members of CHCs were directly appointed by local authorities. The close relationship CHCs had with local authorities influenced how they developed. It broadened their interests to include local authority services as well as the NHS. It also politicised them. Local authorities generally appointed CHC members proportionately on party lines, though some made all appointments from the majority political party. This meant that when there were battles over proposed hospital or service closures that the local authority opposed, the CHC was likely to support the local authority. This made it easier for governments who did not like what CHCs said to discredit them, but it also made them harder to abolish because of their campaigning networks.

CHCs and the public – 'a one sided love affair'

CHCs took the role of representing the public interest seriously. One of the first tasks which CHCs set themselves in 1975 was to make their existence known. Posters were prepared, leaflets distributed and advertisements put in the local press. The public were invited to attend CHC meetings, staff and members addressed local groups. Some CHCs ran stalls at local fetes and produced carrier bags, balloons, bookmarks and beer mats advertising the CHC. The response was disappointing. Most CHCs felt that they were being ignored by the communities which they were supposed to represent in spite of the eagerness and energy that they put into their attempts to reach them. Despite the diversity among CHCs, one theme that runs through all the early annual reports is a lament about '*the frustrating, disappointingly one-sided love affair which CHCs had with the public*' (Klein and Lewis, 1976: 116).

It was perhaps naïve to expect anything else. In the case of the NHS most people were satisfied most of the time and there was no reason to expect them to pay attention to the activities of CHCs on a routine basis. For CHCs there then seemed to be two ways to attract public attention. The first was to provide a specific service to the public, such as information and advice about local health services and support and advocacy for complainants (see Chapter 6). Another was to provide a platform for community or group grievances or associate itself with a popular local issue, which could lead to confrontation with NHS managers. CHCs experimented with many different ways of accessing their communities, including setting up locality forums in rural areas. Members of the public who were interested in commenting on plans and proposals were recruited to health panels, giving the CHC members access to wider views and identifying new areas for further research (Hogg, 1986). Surveys became an important way of finding out what people thought and CHCs derived their legitimacy from these (see Box 5.1).

Consultations

From 1974 health authorities were required to consult CHCs about any closure, substantial variation of use or service development and give them

---

Box 5.1   CHCs and surveys

Though some patients' groups had carried out surveys, CHCs were the first to introduce surveys to the NHS systematically.

Surveys were an alternative source of information for CHCs and they could draw information from members of the public, complaints, community groups, voluntary organisations, individual NHS staff, trade unions and other CHCs.

In the first two or three years, three out of four CHCs had carried out surveys of local services. In 1980 three-quarters had carried out at least one survey in the last three years, generally in order to get information that highlighted needs and gaps in services.

The Royal Commission in 1979 recommended that CHCs be given more resources so they could assess local health issues more effectively. Some patient and public involvement (PPI) forums carried on this tradition, in spite of their more limited resources.

Source: CHC News, 'CHCs at Work', No. 26, December 1977: 6–7.

---

three months to comment and produce counter-proposals if they opposed the closure. In the event of a disagreement, CHCs had the right to appeal to the regional health authority and the Secretary of State. CHCs had been given this right to be consulted in order to encourage health authorities to work with CHCs and speed up the process of change. In the early days it seemed that this was happening. David Owen, the Minister who oversaw the establishment of CHCs, was optimistic that CHCs would be rational and assist in making difficult decisions about cuts and reallocation of resources. '*Meanwhile district management teams are increasingly finding that their community health councils are one of their staunchest supporters. The decision to allow closures of hospitals to take place if CHCs and the AHA and RHA all agreed, was much criticised. It was said that the councils would never agree to any closure: yet, up and down the country, community health councils are agreeing*' (Owen, 1976: 23).

The actual power of CHCs was limited in practice to causing delay and inconvenience. When cuts in public spending were introduced, tensions increased. Hospital closures raise passions among local people and giving CHCs this role in relation to closures encouraged confrontation. Even if CHC members felt the plans were right, it was sometimes hard to stand up against the weight of public opinion, and it was questionable whether, as community representatives, they should. If they 'sided' with management, they might be accused of colluding with them and not protecting local interests.

Some CHCs used their consultation rights to bring about major changes (see Box 5.2) . However, some CHCs felt that their consultation rights had actually weakened rather than strengthened their voice in the NHS. Opposing closures and drawing up alternatives was not rewarding, and it left little time for other activities where the CHC might have had a longer-term impact on the community (Hogg, 1986). A CHC Secretary explained this: '*The*

Box 5.2   Results of consultations

CHCs achieved some striking results where they prepared counter-proposals as a basis for negotiation for developing new services in the community.

- The community hospital in St Mary's Harrow Road and the Lambeth Community Care Centre resulted from plans to extend teaching hospitals at St Mary's Paddington and Lambeth.
- A new GP practice was placed in an underused child health clinic in West Berkshire that the Health Authority wanted to close.

Source: Hogg, 1987.

---

introduction of a formal consultation procedure has ensured that these battles take place on ground which is familiar to health service managers but alien to most local people – including CHC members.... Critics of CHCs have argued that they are not an antidote to the NHS management but an essential part of it – channelling potentially disruptive dissent into manageable forms'.[1] The three-month consultation period for the CHC to comment on proposals was politically convenient for Ministers. *'Ministers could stand outside the political wrangling, while CHCs acted as the lightning rod. This gave the Minister time to consider the political ramifications'* (Winkler, 1989: 8). This enabled hospitals to be closed with a minimum political damage.

Even less rewarding were the procedural battles. Consultation is capable of many interpretations – ranging from a formal process of seeking views about decisions already taken to involvement in the deliberations leading up to the decisions. Many of the disputes in the 1970s were about procedure, where the CHC complained that consultation had not been adequately carried out. CHCs were not legal entities and could not take legal action themselves, but in London three local councils, Brent, Lewisham, and Islington, took legal action on behalf of their CHC to enforce their right to be consulted.

CHCs added a further layer of complexity for those involved in decision-making. This did not mean they were irrational or obstructive in their opposition but consultation takes time and more open administration may also be slower. In 1985 new regulations removed CHCs' power to delay closures. The district health authority could now make a decision without consultation if it was satisfied that it was in the interests of the health service (DHSS, 1985). The CHC still had the right to be consulted after the event, but this became less relevant after 1990 when decisions to close services or hospitals were made by NHS trusts as a result of commissioning decisions made by health authorities. CHCs had no formal relationship with providers and trusts did not have to consult. Informal consultation depended on the willingness of the NHS to consult.

CHCs were abolished in 2003 and patients' forums that replaced them were not expected to address the democratic deficit. Overview and scrutiny committees took over the powers on consultation that CHCs had had. CHCs had been very important in the 1970s when the NHS was inward looking, but as the NHS developed more direct contact with its patients and public, mediating organisations such as CHCs and PPI forums came to be seen as a barrier to involvement rather than enabling it.

Local voices

The introduction of general management in 1983 encouraged managers to relate directly to their consumers and undertake consumer surveys (DHSS, 1983). However, the real impetus came with the introduction of the market in 1990 and the publication of *Local Voices* in 1992. Health authorities were now portrayed as 'champions of the people' (NHSME, 1992). It recognised that there were many different 'voices' and suggested that health authorities should develop long-term relationships with their community and the voluntary sector, rather than relying on one-off consultations. CHCs had lost their monopoly in speaking for their local communities on health matters.

In the 1990s health authorities and trusts up and down the country began to experiment with ways of involving the public such as health panels, population surveys, rapid appraisal, patient satisfaction surveys, consumer audit, critical incident techniques, focus groups, community meetings, consensus conferences, public meetings, opinion polls, and referenda. In Somerset, for example, the health authority set up a rolling programme of focus groups, called health panels, that operated from 1994 until 2003. Sometimes health authorities and trusts bypassed CHCs. Others saw CHCs as a useful ally. CHCs could either work with providers or exercise their independence with the potential for confrontation. Managers attitudes to people who took part also varied (see Box 5.3).

The voluntary sector was offered a new and more prominent role as the authentic representatives of the public. Voluntary organisations were now in demand to legitimate consultations by local authorities and the NHS. When governments in the 1980s had sought to undermine CHCs, they looked to the voluntary sector as an alternative to dealing with CHCs. In 1984 voluntary organisations were given the right to elect three members to joint consultative committees, which were the main forum for the NHS and local authority to plan services jointly. CHCs were ignored though almost half already had observer status on them (DHSS, 1984). The voluntary sector saw their role as complementing that of the CHC who provided information and advice in analysing the issues under discussion (NCVO, 1986).

The number of user-led voluntary organisations grew in the 1980s and 1990s. These groups, pioneered by people with disabilities, mental health service users and people living with HIV, saw traditional voluntary organisations as compromised and paternalistic. They gained their legitimacy from personal experiences of illness or disability and used this to challenge clinical knowledge. Organisations that have been set up by users and those set up by professionals and carers often have different views and understanding of issues of power and its redistribution. Users felt that the way that a disease or

Box 5.3   Managers' attitudes to users

A study found that purchasers tended to divide people who got involved into four categories.

	Possible characteristics	Likely contribution to the service
Naïve user	Members of the public/person on the street Focus on own experience Opinions not informed by professional knowledge Anecdotal experience	Answers questionnaires and surveys Recruited to focus groups/users helpline
Professional user	Involved in several aspects of healthcare 'Gratitude factor' May identify with professional staff and their interests Too close to providers Health service enthusiast	Fund-raising Volunteering League of Friends Available for committees, planning groups, events
Vested interest user	May have long experience of healthcare Long-term user Some particularly bad experience Axe to grind Commitment to change or to improve a particular aspect of the service	Campaigning and lobbying Letters to press and media Frequent contact with service Uses public meetings, consultations, etc. to raise relevant issues Alternative research to make case for change
Informed user	Active in a range of community activities and strong links Sense of public service/duty Other responsibilities allow flexibility Interest, enthusiasm and confidence Proactive in becoming informed	Acts as representative on planning and project groups Gets involved in a range of activities in the service Invited to contribute to conferences, workshops, training events, etc.

- The 'naïve user' was typically viewed as the 'real' or 'authentic' user whose views were particularly valued and sought.
- 'Professional' and 'vested interest' users had long standing relationships or experience with the service and were treated with suspicion.
- Consumers themselves were aware of these different labels and that the label depended more on the attitude and level of understanding of the manager than anything else. Some reported that they were described by all these labels by different managers even within the same organisation, often within a single encounter! For many consumers the need to continually establish and maintain credibility as a legitimate 'voice' was a source of constant anxiety.

Source: Lupton et al., 1998: 118.

condition was defined by medical orthodoxy determined the treatment available to them (Beresford, 2002). In the 1980s there had been major changes in the mental health system. With care in the community those diagnosed as mentally ill became more visible and more vocal. New disciplines were coming into mental health services, creating uncertainty among psychiatrists who had developed their skills in the old asylums. After 1985 patients councils and mental health advocacy projects began to develop. Mental health service users began to describe themselves as 'survivors' of the system rather than patients or consumers (Peck and Barker, 1997). In 1985 there were about a dozen independent survivor-led action groups and by 1995 this had risen to over 350 local, regional and national groups (Campbell, 1996). Some CHCs were instrumental in helping set up user groups.

For the NHS collaboration with the voluntary and community sector was shown to be an effective route to building community relationships and achieving public involvement for the NHS, according to research studies commissioned by the Department of Health (Farrell, 2004). The emphasis on partnership opens up new opportunities for voluntary and community organisations, who may have been outsiders in the policy process. But it also generates new dilemmas as organisations strive to maintain their autonomy while increasingly operating as insiders (Craig et al., 2004). But it was also a burden in terms of time and effort for the voluntary sector. Participating in consultations can dissipate energies for only questionable returns for service users (Barnes, 1999).

Citizens juries

CHCs in the 1970s, citizens' juries in the 1990s and PPI forums in 2003 were all based on models of deliberative democracy. There are three advantages claimed for deliberative democracy. First, that it leads to better quality decision-making by bringing different views into the debate, and increasing the chance that the full implications of decisions will be better understood. The second advantage is for the individual citizen. People who take part develop new skills, have increased self esteem and are more likely to take part in other civic activities afterwards. The third advantage claimed is that there will be enhanced legitimacy and greater public acceptance of controversial decisions.

Citizens' juries met with much interest in the 1990s – they were even described as '*a remarkable experiment in democratic practice*' (Coote and Lenaghan, 1997: 1). The Institute for Public Policy Research was the first organisation to carry out research into citizens' juries and to pioneer the idea in the UK. They defined a citizens' jury as comprising 12 to 16 jurors who were ordinary citizens recruited using a combination of random and stratified sampling with the purpose of being broadly representative of their community. While their main aim was to address an important question about policy or planning, receiving information from independent witnesses, they were primarily advisory and the verdict did not need be either unanimous or binding.

Citizens' juries are based on the belief, that given time and information, ordinary people can make complex decisions about issues that affect them and that this is a better and more unbiased way of obtaining information than, for example, through pressure groups or petitions. Health authorities used juries to involve the public in consultations and debates. Pickard (1998) studied two juries that looked at services for severely mentally ill people. Both juries took place over four days including a weekend. She asked what added value citizens' juries had over CHCs since both involved deliberative democracy. She outlined four points of comparison between citizens' juries and CHCs. First, there is the question of legitimacy. With only 15 members juries had fewer members than CHCs. CHCs could claim that their members set out to represent, not themselves, but the interests of local communities. Citizens' juries had no opportunity to consult with the community and draw other views into the deliberations. Attempts for wider representation in the composition of the jury can also be distorted by group dynamics that can undermine deliberation and create unequal opportunities for effective communication. For example, some groups may be more willing to listen to people who talk with confidence, rather than those who question or express doubts or scepticism. Men may be given more status than women and people from minority groups may feel marginalised (Thompson and Hoggett, 2001).

Secondly, there were also questions about how independent citizens' juries were of the health authority that convened them. The health authority chose the question to be examined, selected the members, the witnesses as well as the evidence and information jurors received. Like any method of consultation, it depended on the goodwill of the body that is consulting.

Thirdly, juries were advisory only and had no authority to follow up or enforce their decisions. This was a problem that CHCs had grappled with for years. Pickard observed that the jurors she studied did not feel sufficiently involved even to attend the health authority public meeting which was convened to discuss their findings. Pickard concluded that the model was flawed in terms of accountability. Citizens' juries are disbanded as soon as they have reported and so cannot engage in an ongoing dialogue even with the health authority which appointed them or with the community from whence they were plucked. By contrast their permanency meant that CHCs could be held to account by local communities and the rest of the health service. Pickard concluded that both the flaws and merits of citizens' juries were shared by CHCs. Yet there were important differences, not the least of which was CHCs' ability to maintain an ongoing dialogue with both the public and statutory authorities and the continuity in engaging with the democratic process. CHCs met regularly and had a permanent remit comprising more members than the average citizens' jury, tapping into public opinion over the long-term and in a variety of ways. Finally, there was the question of cost effectiveness. The four days of the citizens' juries were estimated to require around a quarter of the resources that were needed to run the CHC for a whole year.

After the initial interest, the idea of citizens' juries was not much pursued at local level, but emerged again at national level with New Labour (see

---

Box 5.4   NICE's Citizens Council

It was announced in the _NHS Plan_ in 2000 that NICE would have a citizens council whose task would be to advise it on the value judgments that underlie decisions about treatment and health services.

The Council was composed of 30 members who were recruited as individuals to represent a mirror of society. Anyone involved in patient advocacy groups were excluded and NICE wanted a regular turnover of members. Members, once appointed, opposed this because they felt that they were just beginning to feel at ease and understand what they were doing and their term of office was over. This illustrates a feature of 'managed participation' where value is placed on the 'amateur' status of the representative by managers and professionals. Knowledgeable individuals are considered atypical and so unrepresentative of other lay people. They are dismissed as the usual suspects. When the 'amateur' user gains knowledge and confidence, they lose their value to managers and professionals as they are now 'unrepresentative' (Hogg and Williamson, 2001).

The Council met for three days twice a year. It has reported on issues such as clinical need, whether there are circumstances in which age should be taken into account when making decisions and whether the NHS should pay for drugs to treat very rare diseases. NICE did not necessarily like some of the conclusions. For example, the Council were not in favour of refusing treatment to people with self induced illness.

On the question of whether age should affect the availability of treatment, the Council concluded that no priority should be given to some ages more than to others. They rejected the 'fair innings' argument which would give priority to younger people rather than older people who had had their 'innings'. This was not the result NICE wanted and so they conducted an opinion poll to test this – which came up with a different answer. Rather than spend £150,000 which each Council meeting cost, some members of the NICE steering committee felt it would be more cost effective to undertake opinion polls for £6,000 instead (Davies et al., 2005).

Some Council members had the feeling that they were being used to legitimise rationing. However they did not help NICE in this. The evaluators described the relationship between NICE and the Council thus: _'for NICE the relationship with the Council, as it would be for any host organisation, was rather like that between a set of 'dangerous' animals and their trainers'_ (Davies et al., 2005: 171).

Responsibility for the Citizens Council was transferred to the research and development programme and is now positioned as one of a number of research projects that explore societal values.

Sources: Davies et al., 2005; 2006.

Box 5.4). In July 2007 the new Prime Minister Gordon Brown proposed in Parliament new rights for the British people to be consulted through mechanisms such as citizens juries on major decisions affecting their lives. Spending by government on these consultations was considerable, but there were increasing concerns that such mechanisms are open to manipulation.[2]

Local authorities and involvement

While the NHS had had their own external arrangements to promote participation with CHCs, local authorities managed their own consultations. As local councillors were directly elected, there was not the same imperative to increase democratic engagement. User involvement in local government was encouraged by innovative social service departments but was not a statutory requirement. Though providing services to the same population, the NHS and local government consulted local people separately and in different ways. This changed with the NHS and Community Care Act 1990 that required local authorities to publish community care plans, where possible, jointly with the health authority. For the first time local authorities had a statutory obligation to consult with organisations representing users, carers and voluntary sector providers as well as other agencies. This was 11 years before the duty to consult was given to NHS bodies under Section 11 of the Health and Social Care Act 2001.

Local authorities tried out new ways of consulting users. Newman and colleagues (2002) in a study of two cities found many forums existed: some based on neighbourhoods, some on issues (such as local Agenda 21 groups) devoted to the environment) and some on presumed communities of identity (such as senior citizens and youth). Other initiatives cut across categories, such as those for minority ethnic groups or gay and lesbian groups. Consultation with users and the public was a mandatory part of Best Value reviews, established following the election in 1997 when compulsory competitive tendering was replaced with a new duty for local authorities to ensure best value for the public (Martin et al., 2001). Much local authority consultation was 'consumerist' – that is based on service users rather than citizens. However, different forms of consultation and deliberative methods were used. In a sur-vey two-thirds of local authorities indicated that their experience of participation initiatives was largely positive, but one-third emphasised a negative effect (Lowndes et al., 2001a). They were concerned that participation encouraged unrealistic public expectations, particularly where public demands went against broader local authority policy. Consultation delayed decision-making and some were also concerned that issues could be captured by a particular group, who were not representative of the wider community, leading to populism and short-term decision-making among elected members.

The same researchers also looked at how citizens saw participation. From people's accounts of their own experiences, involvement with the council was largely reactive, a personal reaction to a decision or action that affected them or other local residents. It seems that people like the idea of being able to participate, rather than actually participating. The researchers found that the biggest deterrent to participation was seen to be the lack of council response to the consultation – participation had to be seen to make a difference to be worthwhile. The researchers, however, felt that there was a latent interest among citizens in opportunities for participation into which local authorities need to tap (Lowndes et al., 2001b).

Consultations carried out were generally a process managed by the local authority. The terms of engagement are set by the local authority and people expected to learn the rules of the game and follow them. The views they receive can be controlled. In local government public participation is permissible if the council initiates and controls it. Participation that occurs outside these boundaries is likely to be met with resistance and the labelling of participants as unrepresentative community activists (Crow, 2002).

Some users' views and accounts of personal experiences can be disconcerting. For example, psychiatrists may find it uncomfortable listening to survivors describing their experiences of the psychiatric system as one of having their rights abused (Barnes, 2002). With the new consumerist agenda voluntary organisations faced dilemmas in deciding the extent to which they should respond to the official agenda which was often based on the medical model or pursue their own broader priorities. As Peter Campbell (1996: 224) points out: '*Mad persons as empowered consumers of services and mad persons as equal citizens are two quite different propositions. Outside the health service they are not held in high regard; arguably they are more likely to be seen as dangerous and inferior. There may be a choice between changing services and changing society*'.

Peter Beresford (2002) argues that it is campaigning by the user movement that has made a difference rather than participating in activities offered by statutory authorities. For example, while the Disability Discrimination Act and the Disability Rights Commission fall short of the demands of the disabled people's movement, they provide a framework for highlighting and protecting the rights of disabled people. These were achieved by campaigning, not 'partnerships'.

Overview and scrutiny committees

The last attempt to overcome the democratic deficit was giving local authorities a role in scrutinising the NHS. With the Local Government Act 2000, local authority OSCs replaced the committee system that had operated in local government for over 100 years. Councillors, who were not on the executive, now had the role of representing their constituents and monitoring the executive.

In the *NHS Plan* in 2000 the Department of Health proposed that local authority OSCs should take over the scrutiny function of CHCs. This was seen as a step towards tackling the democratic deficit in the NHS since power was to be transferred from '*unelected community health councils to the all-party scrutiny committees of elected local authorities*' (DH, 2000: 10.27). This arose from two coincidental policies – the reform of local government and the abolition of CHCs. The Health and Social Care Act 2001 enabled authorities with responsibility for social services to review and scrutinise health service matters, and to make reports and recommendations to NHS bodies. They can initiate their own reviews of any topic that affects the health and well-being of local residents. Health scrutiny committees do not have rights of access to NHS premises, but were given powers to summon officers of health trusts to committee meetings, require information from NHS bodies on the planning and provision of health services, and be consulted by health trusts about significant changes to services. NHS bodies are under a duty to respond to committee reports and recommendations, but not bound to accept recommendations.

OSCs took over the right that CHCs had to appeal against a local decision to the Secretary of State for Health. A separate Independent Reconfiguration Panel was set up in 2003 to provide advice to the Secretary of State on contested proposals. The Secretary of State had discretion whether to refer disputed decisions to the panel and this restricted the panel's role. So far there have been few changes as a result. From October 2004 to October 2006, OSCs referred 17 proposals for change to the health secretary. In the majority of cases the Department of Health supported the local NHS proposals. Only three were referred to the reconfiguration panel, which was asked to act as a broker in one further instance (Day and Klein, 2007). The House of Commons Health Committee (2007: 5) was concerned at the readiness of the Secretary of State to intervene, often after a full consultation had been undertaken. They noted that this was threatening to undermine public confidence in the consultation process and recommended that she should refer all cases to the Independent Reconfiguration Panel before intervening.

Health scrutiny was seen as a way of increasing local democracy, accountability and transparency in local health services. At the beginning many had feared that the scrutiny function might have an adverse effect on relationships between local government and the NHS. In fact scrutiny seems to have been successful in promoting closer working between local authorities and the NHS. OSCs have taken a collaborative approach, choosing subjects that cut across health and social care, such as asthma, alcohol misuse or mental health and avoiding subjects for scrutiny that are controversial. It made local authorities more aware of their contribution to their population's health and improved their understanding of health inequalities (Campbell, 2005). In practice, the effect of scrutiny may be to give priority to changes already in the pipeline and needs already recognised, rather than leading to any major change in policy direction.

While OSCs perform a useful function, it is questionable whether this is increasing either democratic participation or accountability (Sandford, 2005). OSCs have limited powers and can only give a limited public accountability for the actions of the external NHS management. However, as they develop confidence and experience in their role, they may be more effective in requiring primary care trusts (PCTs) to be more transparent and compel them to justify their decisions. However, where PCTs maintain that they have to follow national priorities there is nothing the OSC can do (Day and Klein, 2007).

Mainstreaming participation

Overall *Local Voices* did not bring long-term change in the relationship of the NHS and the public. Health authorities still carried out one-off consultations that were confined to fringe issues. Where local people's views conflicted with those of health professionals, they tended to be over-ridden (Cooper et al., 1996). Other case studies on consultation felt that the NHS was not always transparent and honest in its approach to consultation, which lost public trust in both the integrity of NHS managers and the NHS (Peck, 1998). In 1997 the Labour Government saw patient and public involvement as a way to rebuild public confidence in the NHS, and the White Paper, *The New NHS – Modern Dependable* (1997), placed patients and public involvement under this heading rather than democracy or accountability. The *New NHS* did not attempt to increase accountability downwards towards the public. Primary care groups and trusts were only required to be accountable upwards to the health authority. Professional accountability was emphasised which is essentially accountability to peers rather than to the public.

Thinking around patient and public involvement as outlined in the *NHS Plan* was not about democracy, but about mainstreaming – putting patients, not citizens, at the heart of decision-making. This was to be achieved with the new patients' forums and by giving the NHS a duty to consult. During the life of CHCs there had been a debate about whether it was enough for the NHS to consult the CHC and expect them to organise public consultations or whether the NHS should undertake consultations themselves. Section 11 of the Health and Social Care Act 2001 ended this debate and gave NHS bodies a duty to consult.

Participation was also required in other areas, for example to get funding or meet the criteria for NHS foundation trust status. The Department of Health (2003c) gave guidance on many ways that the NHS could consult: complaints schemes, service satisfaction surveys, opinion polls, interactive web sites, citizens panels, co-option to scrutiny committees, question and answer sessions with the public; consultation documents; public meetings, citizens' forums, focus groups, visioning exercises, service user forums, issue forums, shared interest forums, area/neighbourhood forums' and user management of services.

An unintended result of Section 11 and the abolition of CHCs was more confusion about what consultation meant. With CHCs there had been a legal distinction between formal and informal consultation. Even if local people did not understand this, CHCs and the NHS did (see Box 5.5). In time the distinction between consumer surveys and consultation became blurred and the *NHS Plan* in 2000 saw community surveys as a part of consultation and strengthening accountability. The Labour Government announced a systematic national survey in 1997 which aimed to provide regular and comparable information on patients' experiences at health authority and national level (DH, 1997). In the *NHS Plan* it was announced that all trusts would be required to publish the ratings they received from the annual surveys. The responsibility for the national survey then transferred to the Healthcare Commission. However, national surveys are costly and of limited value since improvements can only be made a local level. A crucial question is how the information can be used to achieve change. The strength of surveys carried out by CHCs and patients' forums was that they were in a position to publicise the results and put pressure on local managers to implement the findings.

Box 5.5   What is meant by 'consultation'?

A study of black and ethnic minority groups in Kensington and Chelsea and Westminster found that many organisations were confused by the word 'consultation'.

They reported that they had taken part in consultations where it transpired that many were in fact referring to workshops that provided information about health issues and health prevention. PCTs and NHS trusts did not keep records of public consultations or make clear distinctions between what constituted a consultation and what was an information-giving session. It was therefore not possible to assess the effectiveness of particular consultations.

Source: BME Health Forum, 2006.

At this time managers were concerned that they had to deliver upwards to the Department of Health. Patient and public involvement tended to be positioned in the public relations departments of trusts with the communication functions, whose main task was to negate bad stories (see Box 5.6). It was not seen as part of decision-making. Many tried to involve the public and failed, and found that there were no recriminations if they did not undertake patient and public involvement. The Commission for Health Improvement found that many trusts wanted to support patient and public involvement but did not know how and so patient and public involvement did not become a part of everyday practice in the NHS (CHI, 2004). A review of patient and public involvement in PCTs in London found that public involvement was chronically under-funded, with the focus on short-term initiatives rather than longer-term support (Anderson and Florin, 2000). The consistent theme was the attempts to turn participation into a tool of management. Harrison and Mort (1998) concluded that despite positive attitudes, managers and professionals were careful to leave themselves with ammunition to ignore the outcomes of user involvement. PCTs found that the incentives to undertake good

---

Box 5.6   Where does user involvement fit in the NHS?

The type of user involvement that was undertaken by the NHS depended on where the responsibility was located.

• If the public relations department had responsibility, it focussed on giving out information to the public.
• Public health departments were more likely to work with community-based groups.
• Quality assurance departments favoured surveys and market-based approaches.

However, the same barriers to involvement remained. Managers wanted to control the process and professionals wanted to retain power over the services they provided.

Source: Lupton et al., 1998.

patient and public involvement were not sufficient. A survey by the Picker Institute found that less than half PCTs responding had engaged people in commissioning in the previous 12 months. It concluded that there was a widespread deficit in skills, experience and confidence in carrying out public involvement in PCTs (Chisholm et al., 2007).

The National Health Service Act 2006 replaced Section 11 of the Health and Social Care Act 2001 with Section 242. The Local Government and Public Involvement Act 2007 aimed to clarify consultation by requiring those commissioning services only to consult on 'significant' changes. This meant that there was a duty to consult only where there were proposed changes in the manner of delivery or the range of services to be provided. Many in the user movement felt that this was a dilution rather than an enhancement of the duty to consult. It excludes consultation about funding initiatives, such as the Private Finance Initiative, and probably also decisions to outsource local services, such as the judicial review that Pam Smith took against North East Derbyshire PCT, see Box 5.7. There are also questions about whether local NHS bodies can realistically consult about plans for closures or changes in services which have to be made to meet financial targets or to pay for major reconfigurations of services, under the Private Finance Initiative (PFI). Though these decisions are not a part of the remit for organisations representing patients, they are crucial for citizens.

Conclusions

There had been a long search to overcome the democratic deficit in the NHS, initially through CHCs, then by encouraging NHS bodies to relate directly to their own communities and then through OSCs. With all NHS bodies having

---

Box 5.7   Challenging Section 11

Pam Smith, a patient who was also a parish councillor, applied for a judicial review of the way that North Eastern Derbyshire PCT awarded a general medical services contract to United Health Care without formal consultation. The judge considered that the PCT should have consulted the public under Section 11 of the Health and Social Care Act. However, he threw out the case because the tendering process had been fair and Pam Smith had not raised the matter with her local PPI forum. This was overturned on appeal where it was ruled that the PCT could not avoid its duty to consult.

In another case a former nurse took action about two inpatient wards at Altrincham General Hospital in March 2006 that were closed on the grounds they were no longer safe and the Trust was forced to carry out a proper consultation into the closure.

Source: Sophia Arie, Derbyshire Village wins court battle, *British Medical Journal,* 333: 261; 2 September 2006. Ex-nurse wins wards legal battle 22 September 2006 http:// news.bbc.co.uk/1/hi/england/manchester/5370376.stm, accessed 15 November 2007.

a duty to consult it seemed that there was no further need for a mediating role between the public and NHS managers. Peter Beresford (2002) identifies two approaches: the consumerist approach and the democratic approach.

- The consumerist approach to empowerment is service-centred and concerned to meet the needs of the service, rather than users. This sets limited terms of engagement that may not reflect the real interests of users. They may be invited to have a say or be involved in the running of welfare services that they may not wish to actually receive.
- The democratic approach is people-centred and concerned with rights and needs. For many people with disabilities the issues that concern them are how they can have access to the mainstream – jobs, recreation, environment, transport and non-discrimination. The bottom line, he suggests, is where cash is spent, who is involved, what the redistribution of power is, if any, and how participation helps people make use of services and safeguards their rights.

In practice mainstreaming public participation has led to increased management control of the processes of participation and focusses on consumer rather than democratic issues. The search for the solution to the problem of the democratic deficit was based on the premises that representative democracy embodied by elected representatives was the ideal and sufficient to give legitimacy and accountability for public services. However, as disillusionment grew with representative democracy, the search moved on to looking at broader issues of how democracy might be renewed though greater citizen engagement at local level. This is discussed in Chapter 10.

The Rise of Consumer Rights

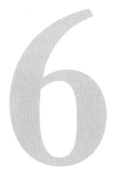

'What is it about choice in health care? Like a child in a sweet shop, we can't resist the offer, even though we know too much may make you sick. The trouble is that choice comes with too much baggage. For the government, it is a way to show voters support for the NHS and the Trojan horse to the professional and organisational cartel. For the citizen, it is the currency by which we calibrate how we have been treated. And for the Economist, it is proof that even those in pain and distress are still able to discharge their essential duties to the market.' Paul Hodgkin, 2005.

Overview

This chapter looks at the impact of the rise of consumerism in the 1980s and 1990s on health policy, equity and collective approaches to participation.

- Consumerism, autonomy and choice were first promoted by the user movement who wanted choice and to be treated with respect and dignity.
- The user movement pioneered advocacy, charters and the provision of consumer information and advice.
- Consumerism and choice were adopted as a management tool by governments to introduce competition and promote the market.
- Consumerism increases inequalities and undermines citizenship by encouraging individuals to act in their own interest and undermines collective approaches to participation based in social rights.

Introduction

User groups since the 1960s questioned how the NHS treated some people, in particular women, people with long-term conditions and black people. They wanted more autonomy, respect and the right to choose. The New Right took this up as evidence of the failure of social rights. They claimed that social rights had failed to achieve equality because:

- People are unequal and there will always be inequalities;
- Increased public spending on welfare and benefits had undermined the wealth-creating private sector; and
- Raised expectations among the poor which are not met, lead to social instability.

The New Right wanted to redefine the relationship of the citizen and the state. In place of the citizen with entitlements and a commitment to public service, they wanted active citizens and citizen-consumers, empowered by property ownership. This approach defines the citizen in narrow terms without reference to politics and collective consultations on policies (Faulks, 1998). However, people need time and money to participate, so this leads to a division of active and passive citizens.

With the market in the 1990s patients and citizens were promoted as consumers. Patients had long been educated to be passive and compliant but they were now to be turned into consumers who would use their power to change and improve services by rewarding good services and penalising poor services. Individuals, sceptical of expert knowledge and acting in their own interests to get the 'best buy' for themselves, would be more effective at maintaining standards than collective decision-making. The key difference between consumers and patients is that consumers are expected to exercise choice. Though the Conservative Government set up conditions for the market, the real initiatives to provide choice came with the Labour Government after 1997. A key objective of choice was to enhance equity by making available to all, what used to only be available to those who could afford it (DH, 2003a).

Information, advice and advocacy

Consumers need information to inform their decisions. Information can give people confidence to question treatments offered and professional advice. Some doctors may find this threatening, while others feel that better informed patients may be more likely to do what they are told. In the 1970s information on services and rights was hard to find and, though it was not a statutory duty, CHCs were encouraged to provide information and advice to the public and support complainants. CHCs pioneered providing independent health consumer information. They produced local directories and guides to using health services and some also guides to private nursing homes and local authority services. Most CHCs saw giving information and advice and acting as a 'patient's friend' as a practical way of advertising themselves to the public. They provided information and advice to the public by phone and face-to-face, including evening surgeries. For this, many wanted accessible high street shop fronts.

With the introduction of the market, providing consumer information had two purposes in government policy: one was to give consumers the information to make choices (where they existed) and the other to force providers to work in different ways through publicity. The *NHS Plan* announced new ways that information would be available to the public with a telephone helpline and website, NHS Direct, that would provide guidance to patients with a health worry and advise them whether to go to the doctor. NHS Direct also operates in Wales and NHS 24 in Scotland. League tables were introduced to rate the performance of hospitals. The Internet also provided new sources of information, giving both public and clinicians the opportunity to access the same information. Some information is evidence-based, but other information is questionable product advertising. There are websites where patients can share their experiences and advise each other. People can use interactive programmes to help them make decisions. Health technology may be very helpful for some people, but will create a new group of excluded people who do not have access to the internet and will include the most vulnerable – older people, people whose first language is not English, who are illiterate and those on low incomes. Access to information that health professionals write about you is also important (see Box 6.1).

Box 6.1   Access to records

Access to health records is also crucial to the consumer. Until 1991 patients did not have the right to see their medical records. The Access to Health Records Act 1990 gave patients the right to see records made about them after 1991. However, access could be refused and information suppressed in certain circumstances, though these circumstances were reduced with the Data Protection Act 1998. These Acts increased the accuracy of notes and reduced the number of personal remarks made by health professionals that they would not want the patient to see.

The *NHS Plan* in England and *Improving Health in Wales* both announced that by 2004 patients would have the right to receive a copy of any letter written from one professional to another about them (DH, 2000). This was piloted in Wales and it was found that it changed the way many doctors related to their patient. Patients liked receiving copies of letters and staff were generally positive, though it involved extra work for them. The benefits were seen to be greater openness and trust between patients and professionals and better informed patients who were encouraged to look after themselves better. As a result all trusts in Wales were required to have policies and procedures by March 2007 (Welsh Assembly Government, 2006).

The introduction of the electronic patient record was also included in the *NHS Plan*. The record would be comprehensive, accessible to patients and healthcare professionals wherever they were. The ownership of confidential information will be particularly important where records are electronic and part of a database that both government and business will want to use. The vision of a patient-owned web record is one that some clinicians welcome, believing that it will empower patients (Muir Gray, 2002). Others are not so sure. Protection of electronic records is less secure in the UK than in a number of European jurisdictions (Korff, 2007).

People's understanding of information varies and some people will not benefit from more information. The term 'health literacy' has been coined to describe the ability to understand written health materials and talk to health professionals. Health illiteracy is more common among older people, socially deprived groups and ethnic minorities. People can be given support to help them with the information, but this is costly. In the pilots for the patient choice schemes the level of support to patients was very important in making it work. Transport to take patients to the hospitals of their choice had been provided in the pilots, but neither the support nor transport was rolled out to the wider scheme (Which?, 2005).

Relying on better information to improve people's health may increase inequalities in the access to healthcare since some people will not be able to access their new rights. Advocacy is important to address this. An advocacy movement developed within the voluntary sector in the 1980s, mainly for people with learning disabilities, mental health problems and whose first language was not English. Similar services had been developed in the 1980s by some CHCs, such as the multi-ethnic advocacy project in Hackney maternity services that was set up and managed by City and Hackney CHC.

Complaints advocacy

People wanting to make a complaint often need help. Patients are generally ill and vulnerable, and entering an alien and complex system run according to rules that they may not know or understand. In addition, they may not know what standards they should expect or how to complain; they may feel that complaining will do no good and may get them into trouble. There are particular problems for mental health service users because of the psychoanalytic tradition that discounts and explains away clients' views as symptoms of their illness. As a result patients who complain may be dismissed as manipulative or as displaying signs of the illness. If their carers complain, this too can be dismissed either as guilt or as part of the family dynamics which might be seen as having contributed to the illness in the first place. Complaints procedures in the NHS are outlined in Box 6.2.

Though it was not a statutory duty, guidance suggested that CHCs should act as the 'patient's friend'. Most CHCs provided assistance to complainants and by 1977 about 30 percent of CHCs had helped individuals to present their complaint about family practitioner services at service committee hearings.[1] By 1980 62 percent of CHCs had assisted a complainant at a service committee hearing (Farrell and Adams, 1981). CHC members did not normally get involved with individual complaints. This was done by staff, who had a contractual obligation to respect patient confidentiality. Members normally received reports on issues that arose from complaints.

With the market the consumer is encouraged to 'voice' their dissatisfaction by making a complaint. The number of complaints more than doubled in England between 1982 and 1991. But in the year following the launch of the Patients Charter in 1991, they increased by over 25 percent. Between

---

Box 6.2   Complaints in the NHS

In 1974 there was no national complaints procedure and the would-be complainant was faced with a complex array of procedures. Complainants had no right to see information and there were no standards for investigation of the complaint.

The need for better complaints procedures was recognised in 1969 when a report on the abuse of mentally handicapped patients in Ely Hospital in Cardiff had caused a scandal. Following this, the Davies committee was set up to report on complaints procedures and it published a report in 1974. The report recommended a national code of practice for dealing with suggestions and complaints about hospitals.

In Scotland complaints legislation in 1972 introduced a standardised code for complaints procedures in hospitals. Nothing happened in England until a private members Bill, which became the NHS Complaints Procedure Act 1985, was passed. Hospitals were now required to have a complaints procedure, though no particular standards were specified.

Problems with the NHS complaints procedure became increasingly apparent as the number of complaints increased. Rather than resolving their grievance, the way complaints were handled sometimes made complainants more dissatisfied (DH, 1994b).

A national procedure covering the NHS in England and Wales was introduced in 1996. There were now three stages: local resolution, a review by an independent review panel and an investigation by the Health Service Ombudsman. However, investment in training staff was limited and problems remained. Many people did not want to talk to staff involved with their complaint and this deterred them from complaining. There were also problems in the perceived independence of independent review in hospitals (NCC, 1997).

In 2002 the role of independent review was handed to the newly formed Healthcare Commission in England. Problems remained and there were enormous variations in the way that complaints were handled (Citizens Advice, 2005). The Healthcare Commission received more complaints than anticipated and developed long backlogs.[2] Further changes in the complaints procedure are now planned for England which will merge the disparate procedures for the NHS and social care (DH, 2007a).

There were also changes in Scotland and Wales. In Wales adjustments were made to the 1996 procedure to make the second stage review more independent. In Scotland the Ombudsman took over responsibility for all investigations that were not resolved at local level.

1991 and 1994 complaints to the General Medical Council rose by almost 50 percent.[3] It was clear that the policy to turn the compliant patient into a consumer was having some effect. The increasing workload of CHCs and their insistent demands for more resources, led the DHSS to suggest that CHCs should stop assisting individuals first in 1981 and this was often repeated. It suggested that there were other sources of help available to people who wished to pursue a complaint – personal friends, MPs, local councillors and citizens advice bureaux.

CHCs argued strenuously against this. They found the contact with patients and carers provided by complaints was a useful source of information about how patients actually experienced services and helped them in their scrutiny and representation roles. The Wilson report that reviewed the NHS complaints procedure noted the importance of the CHC's role in supporting complainants (DH, 1994b).The introduction of the new complaints procedure in 1996 led to renewed questions about whether complainants still needed independent support. Others saw helping individuals as an important service. After the abolition of CHCs, Frank Dobson, the first Secretary of State in the 1997 Labour Government, considered that helping complainants was one of the things that CHCs had done well (Gerrard, 2006).

With the abolition of CHCs, the role of 'patient's friend' need to be carried out elsewhere. In the *NHS Plan,* the Department of Health proposed to set up a new patient advocacy and liaison service (PALS) to help patients with problems and to steer patients and families towards the complaints process where necessary. This was based on the model of patient representatives piloted within hospitals in the early 1990s (McIver, 1993).

No provision was made for independent complaints advocacy to replace the service provided by CHCs. It was assumed that PALS could do this. The voluntary sector and CHCs argued that PALS would be employed by the service and so could not be advocates or provide independent advice to complainants. The argument was won and it was recognised that complaints advocacy needed to be independent of the organisation complained about to have credibility with the public. In the NHS and Community Care Act 2001 the Secretary of State was given the duty to ensure independent advocacy services for the people requiring assistance when making complaints. This service was called the independent complaints advocacy service (ICAS). PALS were renamed patient advice and liaison services and were left out of the legislation.

There is little information about how effective PALS and ICAS are. It clearly made sense to have a point of contact in each hospital to help deal with people's problems as they arose, rather than an outside body, such as a CHC. ICAS are able to provide a national service, replacing the patchy service provided by CHCs. But some things have been lost. There are no local offices and so access is harder for the public. CHC staff generally knew the local services and local managers and so could sometimes mediate successfully on individual complaints. CHCs could use the information gained from complaints to monitor local services and follow up to see whether changes had been made as a result of a complaints investigation.

In Wales patient support officers, with a role similar to PALS. CHCs were given additional resources to develop their complaints advocacy role, with several CHCs generally working together to provide the service.

Charters and rights

Healthcare charters were first developed in the USA in the 1970s with the recognition that consumers needed rights and protection in the market. In the

UK the first charters were produced by voluntary organisations for campaigning purposes in the 1980s. These included the charter for the children in hospital produced by NAWCH (now Action for Sick Children) in 1984; the Patients Charter produced by the Association of Community Health Councils for England and Wales (ACHCEW) in 1986; and a Charter for Carers produced by the Carer's Alliance in 1989. These were aspirational charters, but they recognised the tension between the long-term vision of a voluntary organisation and what is achievable and acceptable to health professionals. To be effective charters depend on the support from people with the power to implement them. All these user charters were developed after lengthy consultation with both users and health professionals. Between 1987 and the early 1990s some health authorities set about developing their own charters, generally taking the ACHCEW charter as a base (Hogg, 1994b). The UK was the first country in Europe to adopt a Patients' Charter in 1991 (and subsequently to abolish it). Between 1994 and 2004 nine other European Union states adopted patients' charters (Patients Association, 2005).

The Patient's Charter

In the 1990s the Conservative Government adopted charters as a way of promoting the market and choice (see Box 6.3). In 1991 the Government launched the UK Patient's Charter for acute and community services and later for primary care. The Charter aimed to make the health service more responsive to users by setting out the rights and standards that consumers should expect. These standards provided the basis for the targets that managers were expected to meet. Three new rights were established: the right to detailed information about local health services, to a guaranteed admission to hospital within two years of joining the waiting list, and a prompt and full investigation of any complaint.

Box 6.3   The Citizen's Charter

The Citizen's Charter was launched in 1991. This was a move away from citizenship defined as rights and duties enjoyed by people linked together in a common political purpose. It envisaged a society where citizens are seen as individual consumers in the marketplace. Providers were seen as the problem and the Government with its charter was trying to solve this.

Such charters did not address discrimination or recognise the unequal access that citizens or patients have. Faulks (1998) sees three reasons for the introduction of the Charter.

- The Charter legitimised the restructuring of the public services;
- If the targets set were unrealistic, confidence in public services could be undermined and this would point out the advantages of private services; and
- The Charter enabled the Government to distance itself from the problems of the public sector.

However, the Patient's Charter was introduced with speed and little consultation with staff, managers or users. It was imposed by Downing Street against the wishes of some health ministers (Dyke, 1998). Without asking them, the Government defined the two most important issues for consumers as waiting time and choice. There were many criticisms of the Charter both from the NHS and from patients' groups. For staff the Charter was seen as one-sided. It was a top-down initiative which they saw as a political stick with which to beat them. It distorted priorities in health services as providers tried to meet targets that were not based on clinical need. Staff felt that the Charter raised patients' expectations, often by implying choice where it did not exist and leading to dissatisfaction when the expectations were not met. It put pressure on staff while ignoring patients' responsibilities and engendered a culture of blame. It also encouraged staff to cheat in order to meet the standards. For example, there were instances where patients were transferred from trolleys to chairs simply to comply with the Charter standard for admission to the ward from the accident and emergency department (Farrell et al., 1998).

For patients the Charter was confusing because it muddled rights with aspirations. Many of the 'rights' were not enforceable but were service aspirations that could not always be met. The Charter measured those parts of the process that were easy to measure but not necessarily those most important to patients or to staff, such as clinical outcomes. Charters produced by voluntary organisations, differed in many ways from those produced by the Government. In general, users were more concerned about the boundary between home and hospital and between health and social care. They were concerned with the way the services were provided and whether their autonomy was respected as well as other things that affected their ability to cope with their illness, such as income, housing and childcare. They were concerned about access to services, such as mental health services, where using them may lead to discrimination and even a loss of civil rights (Hogg, 1994b).

Choice helps people feel in control of what is happening to them and is a major part of healing. But choice defined by user groups had a different meaning from choice that operates in the market. It was not choice of hospital or choice of provider that was seen as important. A survey for the Healthcare Commission found that choice about appointment times and hospital referrals was ranked in the lowest 10 percent of a list of 82 patient priorities (Boyd, 2007). Choice of treatments within services is important. For people with disabilities or long-term conditions, choices may be limited and they want services that are responsive to individual preferences and opportunities to choose different treat-ments.

The Patient's Charter was essentially a management tool at a time of organisational change. It was used to inform patients of the services they should expect and even demand, but its primary aim was to impose central government control indirectly over the performance management of trusts in the name of the consumer (Crinson, 1998).

New Labour's NHS Charter

In 1997 the incoming Labour Government promised a new NHS Charter that would include both rights and duties. This was a move away from the simple view of the citizen as consumer to see citizens as having rights that were dependent on fulfilling responsibilities (Jochum et al., 2005). New Labour aimed to promote a reciprocal relationship between the state and citizens, in which citizens become partners. Greg Dyke, who had run London Weekend Television and later became Director General of the BBC, was asked to develop proposals for a new NHS Charter for England. Instead he proposed a different approach. He considered that the failure of the Charter was because it was imposed on local services by the Government and had no local ownership for the standards or what it was trying to achieve. He suggested that the Department of Health should start with a value statement for the NHS that all patients and the NHS could sign up to, covering issues such as fairness, excellence, partnership, communication as well as the importance of patients treating staff with a dignity and respect (Dyke, 1998). The new Charter would shift the emphasis to local services. Local charters would include the national values statement, a list of legally enforceable rights (which are very few), national minimum standards and standards defined nationally but set locally, as well as standards defined and set locally.

Greg Dyke was asked specifically to address the issue of the responsibilities of patients, such as their failure to return hospital equipment, making unnecessary demands on GPs, inappropriate use of accident and emergency services and generally abusive behaviour towards staff. However, he found the situation to be more complex than the Government anticipated. He found some trusts had been successful in reducing the number of patients who did not keep appointments, but these efforts had been abandoned because though they were more efficient, no savings were made. The hard core of patients who act irresponsibly or aggressively were difficult to deal with. He concluded that, without effective sanctions, any concept of patients' responsibilities was meaningless. The ultimate sanction would be to refuse to treat people who acted irresponsibly. However, some of these irresponsible patients would be those most in need of care and refusing to treat them went against the founding principles of the NHS. Treating people who are deemed to be acting irresponsibly is the price to be paid for a free universal service, he concluded.

The Government was not impressed with his low key consensual approach to patients' rights or his reluctance to tackle patients' responsibilities. However, the manifesto commitment to replace the Patient's Charter remained to be honoured and in January 2001 it was replaced with *Your Guide to the NHS*, which provided information on responsible use of health services, tips on healthy living and advice for patients on which services they should access when feeling unwell. However, by 2005 it was not available either in hard copy or even on the Department of Health website.

In Scotland the Patient's Charter was replaced by a package including guides to rights and responsibilities and information on rights produced by the Scottish Consumer Council.

Legal action and the Human Rights Act

The days of charters as a management tool were over. The next charter to impact on the NHS and its relationship with patients was a very different affair. The Human Rights Act 1998 incorporated the European Convention on Human Rights into UK law and came into force in October 2000. The Act makes it unlawful for any public body to act in a way which is incompatible with the Convention, unless the wording of an Act of Parliament means they have no other choice. It does not apply to private sector providers, even if funded by the NHS.

Several articles of the Convention can be used by patients to challenge their treatment – or lack of it – by the NHS. The right to life (Article 2) could be used to demand aggressive treatment, to keep alive patients who doctors thought too ill for resuscitation. Article 3 requires that someone is not subjected to inhuman or degrading treatment, which could be used where patients

---

Box 6.4   The Human Rights Act and commissioning decisions

Legal action by individuals to insist on the continuation of treatment against medical advice have implications for a cash strapped health service.

In 2006 a woman took a judicial review against her primary care trust to force it to fund a new and unlicensed drug for breast cancer, herceptin. The costs of prescribing herceptin were about £24,000 per patient a year. Funding on this scale can only be made by cuts to other cancer services. A team in Norfolk and Norwich University Hospital estimated that they could pay the £2.3 million necessary to fully fund herceptin for 75 patients likely to be eligible, but only if they did not treat 355 patients receiving other cancer treatments or 208 patients receiving chemotherapy (Barrett et al., 2006). Through such publicity breast cancer achieved priority over other cancers, with the result of longer waits for chemotherapy for other, less romanticised cancers.

Charlotte W was born three months prematurely, weighing just 1lb and less than five inches long with severe brain and lung damage. Her parents fought for two years in the courts to force the hospital looking after her to ensure she would be resuscitated, if necessary. The hospital won the first round, then later the parents appealed and it was agreed that doctors should resuscitate the child if necessary. Finally as the baby's condition deteriorated again, the decision was once again left to the doctors. Charlotte survived against the odds and medical opinion, but there was not a happy ending. Though doctors agreed to discharge the baby home with 24 hour care, by then the parents had split up and she remained in hospital and moved eventually to foster care. The costs were estimated at over £110,000 a year and the legal battles a further £500,000. While massive media attention was given to the campaign, little attention was given to the outcome for Charlotte or the costs.[4]

Whatever the ethical perspective, such cases will continue and impact on the other services that can be commissioned. Rationing decisions are about life and death ultimately.

feel that the quality of care was so inadequate that it was degrading. Article 5 – the right to liberty – has implications for psychiatric patients, where the patient is detained without consent. Article 12 gives the right to marry and found a family. This could be used by couples who are having difficulty conceiving and want NHS funded in-vitro fertilisation.

Legal action is increasingly used to try and divert resources towards particular services or individuals, in effect meaning that other people will not receive services because the funding is not available. Patients have used judicial review of the decisions of primary care trusts to refuse to pay for treatment or medication (see Box 6.4). Often legal action is funded by the pharmaceutical industry who have much to gain from wider availability of their new and most expensive drugs.

The problem with individual rights is that they are rarely simple and there is a difficult balance between the rights and responsibilities of citizens and between respect for the individual and the public interest. In practice, the impact on healthcare of the Human Rights Act is likely to be limited. The intention of the Act was to protect citizens from abuse and not to make decisions about the way healthcare is planned and which services are funded.

There may be new possibilities in human rights where they are not seen exclusively as a tool for litigation to check on the abuse of state power, but are used by communities to tackle discrimination and poverty. Human rights should be used as a tool for tackling social injustice, enhancing public services and empowering people to participate fully in society (Ghose and Weir, 2007).

Patients' groups and other interests

It is not just the government who wanted to influence patients to become consumers, professional and commercial interests also see benefits in working with patients groups. Some groups were setup by professionals, while in others users work closely with professionals in partnership and others are user-led. The key issue is the role that users, professionals and others play in their governance. The richest and largest groups tend to be the older groups that were set up by professionals and where professionals remain heavily involved. The relationship that a voluntary organisation has to professionals largely determines the ease with which it can obtain funding, find acceptance with policy-makers and how radical it is in representing patients' interests (see Box 6.5). Health consumer and patients' groups lack economic leverage and their expertise and knowledge are less highly valued than professionals (Baggott, 2007).

There has been a rapid increase in the number of not-for-profit patients' groups. Such groups tend to be organised around specific diseases or conditions and provide a platform from which they can try to influence treatment priorities and services. Increasingly patients' groups see their mission as not simply providing services but in influencing how government prioritises expenditure on medical research, healthcare and public health. They aim to help

---

Box 6.5   Patients groups, professionals and industry

Patients' groups are most powerful when linked with other interests.

Patients' groups aim to influence government and its agents, such as the National Institute for Health and Clinical Excellence (NICE). Patients' groups presented almost as many witnesses before the NICE technology appraisal panel as medical groups and more than the industry. Research on the campaign to make beta interferon available for the use in multiple sclerosis revealed the existence of a network of experts that is linked with patients' groups. Access to this network enabled the Multiple Sclerosis (MS) Society to present expert evidence in addition to the more emotional stories of MS patients. The MS Society was able get media publicity in the media by mobilising its members. (Duckenfield and Rangnekar, 2004).

However, patients groups are likely to be most successful when they work in conjunction with industry. The study found that where industry and patients' groups launched appeals against NICE decisions they had a very high success rate (83 percent) in overturning NICE decisions (Duckenfield and Rangnekar, 2004). The major charities that have campaigned against NICE rulings received funding by the manufacturers of the drug for which they were campaigning.[5]

---

patients get access to new drugs and treatments as well as private and alternative healthcare providers. By 1997 there were 256 in the UK, 54 percent of which were formed after 1980 (Duckenfield and Rangnekar, 2004). Since the mid-1990s the influence of patients' groups has increased. As their budgets grow and staff become more specialised, patients' groups have developed expertise in corporate activities such as communications, fundraising, policy formation, advocacy and research evaluation. These trends are likely to continue and the influence of patients' groups to expand.

Pharmaceutical companies see the benefits of working with patients' groups and using them to market their drugs to consumers. The logic of the market is to cut out the middle person – in this case the health professional. In the long run drug companies aim to bypass medical professionals who are more sceptical or cost-conscious and market themselves directly to the public. Consumer organisations have criticised the industry for its lack of transparency and unscrupulous marketing. They claim that drug companies are adopting new ways to influence consumers, such as sponsoring patients' groups in funding disease awareness campaigns as well as using old methods such as offering hospitality to medical experts or opinion leaders (Consumers International, 2006).

Initially the company may obtain good public relations and advertising by being associated in the minds of patients and professionals with 'feel good' initiatives. In the long-term by supporting voluntary organisations, pharmaceutical companies can create consumer demand for their drugs and exert pressure to fast track new drugs through the licensing procedures. Schering, for example, set up a bogus patients' group – MS Voice – with no patient participants but with a website designed to recruit people to its lobbying campaign. Another pharmaceutical company, Biogenic, set up a campaign 'Access to Action' and purchased advertisements in national newspapers. Complaints from the MS Society persuaded Schering and Biogenic to abandon their campaigns under pressure from the Medicines Control Agency (Duckenfield and Rangnekar, 2004). In spite of the shared interest between patients' groups and commercial companies, many groups fear that they may lose their independence and credibility by being associated with drug companies.

Policies that promote self help and personal responsibility of consumers fit the industry agenda. They argue that *'if payers truly want consumers to take more responsibility for their own health care they should encourage the manufacturers to engage directly with the consumer rather than maintaining the 'Chinese walls' that exist in most countries today'* (Mills, 2000: 4). Direct to the consumer advertising is a right that drug companies already enjoy in the USA and want in Europe. Proposals for a TV channel funded by drug companies to provide information and promote their products is a further example of the trend to market drugs directly to patients and put pressure on providers in this way.[6] Whatever the ethics of direct to consumer advertising, it is unlikely to improve the health of the population as a whole. It is more likely to escalate costs by increasing the demands on public health services by those least in need, thus adding to the problems that it was hoped patients acting as consumer would address.

The implications of the consumer-citizen

Consumerism is attractive to the public compared to the culture of the passive and compliant individual who accepted what was offered and was grateful. Consumerism may deliver some changes in public services, but it puts efficiency before equity and this can lead to inequalities. Choice assumes that all citizens have the resources to be active consumers, which is not true. Inevitably, choice will lead to inequalities because people will not have equal access to the information or the resources to take up their options (Farrington-Douglas and Allen, 2005). For everyone to have an equal opportunity, there will need to be special efforts, which will be expensive (Thorlsby and Turner, 2007). Primary care trusts may find ensuring equitable choice is unaffordable (Bate and Robert, 2005). It can lead to less transparency because secrecy can be justified for commercial reasons. Many commentators point to the steady retreat of the civil ideal in the face of the market. David Marquand (2004) sees this as the chief threat to democracy in Britain today and argues that citizens exerting their rights in the market are incompatible with egalitarianism required for citizenship.

Consumerism is unsatisfactory as a model for two further reasons. First, consumerism does not necessarily improve the patient experience. It can undermine the trust between patients and healthcare professionals (see Box 6.6). Second, relying on the individual consumer to bring about change also undermines collective participation. Services that meet the perceived needs of individual users better may not be the same as those that deliver better public health outcomes, such as morbidity and mortality. The disability movement

---

Box 6.6   Consumerism and the doctor-patient relationship

Consumers need to be sceptical and mistrustful but this is not necessarily beneficial to the therapeutic relationship.

- The relationship between patient and clinician is very personal: mostly it involves a doctor or healthcare worker touching or examining your body, something few experience without some emotion.
- Illness, disease and disability are highly emotional states and make it difficult for people to think like and take the role of a rational and objective consumer engaging in a business transaction.
- The consumerist approach may be counter-productive, undermining the trust and faith that are central to the healing and comfort of ill people who seek medical help (Lupton, 1997).

There are other models that take better account the complexity of the doctor-patient relationship. These are the autonomous patient proposed by Angela Coulter (2002) and the resourceful patient proposed by Dr Muir Gray (2006). Muir Gray argues that the fundamental contract between patient and clinicians in the twenty-first century should start with the assumption that patients are competent and responsible, providing that they are given the resources to exercise their responsibility.

---

argues that those who experience discrimination in housing, education, social situations and personal relationships, want social action to address the causes of discrimination and appropriate support. The right to make a complaint is an important consumer right. However, the complaints process encourages patients to see staff as the source of problems in the NHS, rather than the result of wider policies. In a market individual voices replace the collective approaches to a public voice, based in ideas of social rights. Increasingly it seems that complaints are used to voice concerns about commissioning decisions about the services provided – which would previously have been discussed and debated in the public domain.

The problems of consumerism come into sharp relief when looking at the options available to mental health service users. Mental health services were developed by psychiatrists who felt they knew what users needed. This created a system that most users did not value or feel was appropriate to them. Mental health users may want a choice of different types of services, but they may only be offered medication. They do not all choose to make use of services; some may enter 'voluntarily' because otherwise they would be compulsorily forced to. Many cannot refuse treatment as there are no alternatives or there would be public safety concerns if they did. 'Disruptive' behaviour may lead to the loss of rights. For them using their 'voice' is difficult because professionals are powerful and often see the world from a very different perspective from service users. People from black and ethnic minorities face racism in services that may be institutional to the NHS, as well as the other problems facing mental health service users.

Collective participation and the support of other users may be necessary for vulnerable users and for those who suffer health inequalities to help them express their 'choices'. Bolzan and Gale (2002) looked at two groups of excluded consumers – older people and people with mental health problems. These groups felt themselves to be marginalised and did not see themselves as consumers. They challenged the imposition of the role of consumer and found alternative routes to get their views across, such as participating in arrangements with providers. The researchers concluded that older people and people with mental illness used collective action to educate, empower, lobby and challenge the status quo. They contested the individualistic under-pinning of their status as consumers and asserted the importance of collective action.

Citizenship is a status that demands political participation. Catherine Needham (2003) contrasts the citizen consumer with the participatory citizen (Box 6.7). She argues that treating citizens as consumers has profound impli-cations for the relationship between government and citizens. It restricts citizens to a passive consumption of politics, excluding them from playing a creative and productive role in civic life. In the long run if people are not emotionally involved in the politics of making public services better, they may just demand more and become increasingly dissatisfied. Needham sug-gests that rather than delivering a satisfied pliant citizenry, it will foster priva-tised and resentful citizen-consumers whose expectations cannot be met.

Conclusions

In the 1980s and the 1990s the government and the right hijacked the ideas about consumer rights and charters developed by the user movement. The

---

Box 6.7   Comparison of the citizen-consumer and the participatory citizen

The citizen-consumer	The participatory citizen
Self regarding	Community regarding
Reflexive preferences	Preferences shaped by deliberation
Market accountability	Political accountability
Voice as complaint	Voice as discussion
Loyalty to the political community secured through promotional advertising	Loyalty to the political community based on common citizenship
Instrumental attitude to politics: political activity as a means	Non-instrumental attitude to politics: political activity as an end

Source: Needham, 2003.

government took their calls for more autonomy and choice and translated them into consumer choice. The arguments may sound the same but they start from very different premises.

There is little evidence that the NHS is more patient-centred as a result. A study of national patients surveys 2002–2007 concluded that the most significant problem was the failure of clinical staff to provide active support for patient engagement (Richards and Coulter, 2007). Individual choice is about patterns of private consumption and very different from public choices that are collective decisions about who will receive public services. Arrangements for collective engagement are essential for setting priorities and addressing inequalities that can emerge from market-driven healthcare. Choice cannot replace voice and makes public voice more important not less. There need to be collective ways for citizens to express their voice in order to counter balance the self interest of the consumer. Calnan and Gabe (2001: 124) point out that consumerism is '*unlikely to bring about the significant improvements in the quality of care that might be achieved if the service was made directly accountable to users through community participation in decision-making, in line with local health needs. But this would involve a different view of the citizen as a member of a community, with rights and duties balanced by mutuality and control*'.

Promoting Health

'... the demand for a healthier society is, in itself, the demand for a radically different socio-economic order'.

Lesley Doyal, 1979: 297.

Overview

This chapter looks at the relationships between policies on user involvement, public health and tackling inequalities.

- Public health policies since the mid-1970s have focussed on how individuals can keep themselves healthy and by improving access to healthcare rather than tackling the underlying social and economic determinants of ill health.
- Policies promoting participation must address the wider determinants of health. Policies that focus on self help, choice and changing lifestyles are likely to increase inequalities in health.
- Approaches that work with communities are more likely to increase participation and engagement to those who suffer the poorest health in society.
- Public health policies in future are likely to be aligned with policies on user involvement as part of devolution to neighbourhoods.

Introduction

Many factors influence health: individual factors such as age, sex and genes; how we live; social and community networks and the general socio-economic, cultural and environmental conditions of our lives. In reality the control individuals have over factors that affect their health is limited. It is estimated that over 70 percent of what determines people's health lies in their demographic, social, economic and environmental conditions and outside the domain of health services (House of Commons, 2001: 124). This is illustrated in Box 7.1.

Among the expected, but often implicit, benefits of involving patients and the public is better health for the population. Different perspectives about the

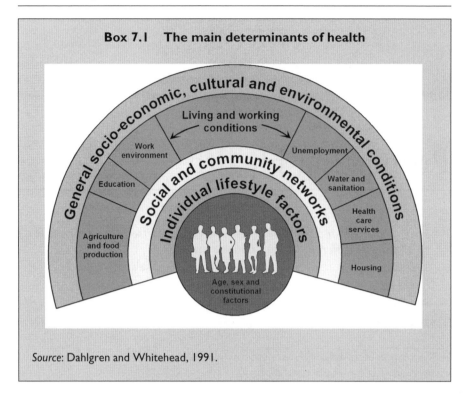

Box 7.1 The main determinants of health

Source: Dahlgren and Whitehead, 1991.

causes of ill health and who should be responsible for public health has led to a fragmentation of public health policy. There are tensions between the different strands of public health policy. Inequalities can be tackled through government interventions, through medical interventions and health education that targets individuals and community development approaches. Each of these approaches envisages a different relationship between the individual and the state. The public health movement was a response to the health crisis caused by industrialisation and the growth of cities. By the end of the nineteenth century the public health movement had branched into two different and competing areas: promoting general improvements in social conditions and preventive medicine promoting specific preventive and curative interventions in the health service, such as health education, screening and immunisation. Responsibility for public health moved from local government to the NHS. With the rise of consumerism self healthcare and choice have been favoured by policy-makers, giving more responsibility to the individual.

However, health may improve for the population generally while inequalities in health between groups increase. This happens when responsibility for health emphasises individual and community lifestyles and ignores social determinants of health, such as business practices and government policy on transport, housing and taxation.

National action and tackling inequalities

Promoting health is complex for governments to take on. It is not straight forward like building roads, schools or hospitals, but about achieving healthier communities, and ensuring that children have the right environment in which to grow and develop. Public health policy requires long-term commitment and interagency collaboration at all levels. Often the long-term needs of health policy are at odds with the short-term pressures of government (Hunter, 2004).

Tackling the wider determinants of health and inequalities requires government action. Poverty, unemployment, crime, poor housing and environmental pollution are influenced by political decisions at national and international level. Only governments can promote health through taxation and regulation. Local authorities, individuals and pressure groups cannot successfully take on commercial vested interests, such as the tobacco, food and drink industries, on their own.

Though the Department of Health has overall responsibility for public health, most of the actions that might reduce inequalities and promote public health are outside its powers. Professional, commercial and other interests continue to dominate public health policy. Promoting gambling may help regenerate poor areas, but is likely to increase gambling and make addiction to gambling an increasingly important public health issue. Alcohol policy has allowed extended opening hours, cheaper alcohol and clusters of pubs in city centres which encourage young people to binge drink. Obesity is newly

---

Box 7.2   Tackling obesity

Obesity increases the risk of chronic disease, such as diabetes, stroke, coronary heart disease, cancer and arthritis. The Government's Foresight project has concluded that Britain has become a country where overweight is the norm. By 2050 it is estimated that 60 percent of adult men and 50 percent of adult women and about 25 percent of children could be obese. The financial impact to society attributable to obesity at current prices is estimated to become an additional £45.5 billion by 2050.

The report recognises that biology and behaviour play a part, but that we live in an 'obesogenic' environment, with an abundance of high energy food, motorised transport and sedentary lifestyles. Just as we had passive smoking, we now have passive obesity. Some people, including the most disadvantaged are especially vulnerable.

The report concludes that policies aimed solely at individuals will be inadequate to reverse this trend. A whole systems approach is needed from the production and promotion of healthy diets to redesigning the built environment to promote walking, together with wider cultural changes to shift societal values around food and activity. It will require actions not only by government, both central and local, but also by industry, communities, families and society as a whole.

Source: Foresight, 2007.

recognised as a major public health problem and the costs of ill health and treating diseases arising from obesity will be great in the future for the NHS, but it cannot act alone (see Box 7.2).

Actions at local level by local authorities, primary care trusts and community groups are likely to be marginal without national direction, backed up with resources. There are limits to what can be achieved by communities.

Public health policies

The public health movement in the nineteenth century aimed to reduce the health damaging consequences of individualism and capitalism by providing sanitation and housing, reducing poverty and pollution and tackling the socio-economic causes of ill health. The movement was led by engineers with little role for lay people. They offered technical solutions to problems but did not have a philosophy about the causes of ill health or the relationship of society and disease that might have provided the basis for a wider movement.

With the establishment of the NHS, local authorities lost responsibility for providing health services but retained public health. In 1974 local authorities lost this also to the NHS. These changes led to the marginalisation of public health. Health authorities with their origins in managing hospitals did not see the relevance of recreation facilities, job creation, food hygiene or accident prevention to health services. Though local authorities were still responsible for social care and housing, sanitation, parks and recreation, they became less aware of the importance of their services for the health of the population.

In the 1970s the government took a new interest in public health, with the endorsement of the Treasury. The aim was to save money spent on healthcare rather than a desire to reorient medical care. Governments were increasingly preoccupied with the funding of the NHS and hoped that prevention might save money in treatment costs in the longer-term (Lewis, 1992). *Prevention and Health: Everybody's Business* was published in 1976. For the first time the Department of Health and Social Security seemed to recognise the wider causes of ill health and the need for a broader approach to tackle them (DHSS, 1976c). It pointed out that curative medicine might be subject to the law of diminishing returns and that the major breakthroughs in promoting health had been due to improvements in clean water, housing and the environment and were well established before screening and immunisation programmes were introduced which, often erroneously, took the credit. In spite of this, the focus was essentially on what individuals could do. Public health was also promoted at national level by a succession of external agencies (see Box 7.3).

In 1977 the Labour Government commissioned a report on inequalities in health – the Black Report (see Box 7.4). This took a broad view of cross-agency action to tackle the broad determinants of health. However, the Conservative Party came to power in 1979 and did not favour state intervention, preferring to see health as an individual responsibility. As the evidence of the increase in health inequalities grew, pressure mounted on the Government to do something to address them. Health inequalities were rediscovered

Box 7.3   Promoting health nationally

In 2005 the National Institute for Clinical Excellence (NICE) merged with the Health Development Agency to form the **National Institute for Health and Clinical Excellence**. For some this seemed to be a take over of public health by an organisation dominated by clinical and pharmaceutical interests. This was the continuation of an old story.

The **Health Development Agency** had itself replaced the Health Education Authority in 2000, as a research-based body to provide evidence for public health.

The **Health Education Authority** was seen by campaigners as still imbued with the health promotion culture of the 1980s that placed responsibility for ill-health firmly with the individual.[1]

In 1987 the Health Education Authority had replaced the **Health Education Council** in England which had made enemies of powerful vested interests and upset some political sensitivities because of its belief that health inequalities were important at a time when government officially denied they existed.

The fears that the transfer of public health to NICE would medicalise it soon seemed to be justified. When NICE published its guidance on health inequalities it was criticised for dealing with public health issues in the context of a national sickness service, without addressing the causes of the diseases. It focussed on the reduction of mortality from cancer and heart disease, and followed the medical model of focussing on interventions, rather than on how different agencies work together (UK PHA, 2007).

Box 7.4   Tackling inequalities in health – the Black Report

The Labour Government convened a Research Working Group in 1977 on inequalities in health with Sir Douglas Black, President of the Royal College of Physicians, as Chair. However, the Group reported to the Conservative Government of Margaret Thatcher who did not share the broadly collectivist view of public health of the previous government.

The report was submitted in 1980 and recommended government intervention to tackle child poverty, free school milk and free school meals, more spending on housing, investment in day care and antenatal facilities and in home help and nursing services for disabled people. It received a frosty reception. Only 260 duplicated copies of the typescript were made available. There was no press release but copies were sent to selected journalists on the Friday before August Bank Holiday. This strategy backfired and one journalist realised the significance and persuaded the Working Group to call an alternative press conference, which was held at the Royal College of Physicians.

The Government was not interested in tackling the social determinants of health that would lead to more public spending and a reaffirmation of the welfare state and social rights. The Black Report, with its weighty research evidence, was a continuing embarrassment for the Government and used by pressure groups and the opposition throughout the 1980s.

Source: Townsend et al, 1988.

in the 1990s as 'health variations'. *The Health of the Nation* was published (DH, 1992). The targets around prevention were narrow and clinical about avoiding premature death rather than promoting health in the community. The risk factors considered were individual – smoking, diet and blood pressure. There were achievements for user groups. Mental illness was for the first time recognised as a public health issue and targets for breast and cervical cancer, which were supported by many women's organisations, were set. The report was criticised by the Labour Party because it did not recognise the impact of socioeconomic and environmental factors. *The Health of the Nation* was an important symbol but did not significantly change the behaviour of health authorities because public health targets were less important than other national policies, such as bringing down hospital waiting lists (DH, 1998a; NAO, 1996a). It was also seen as a Department of Health initiative, without cross-departmental support at national level or local government commitment at local level.

In Wales there was a better understanding of the impact of health inequalities on health. The first public health strategy was published in 1989 and focussed on ways of achieving health gain and included strategies for involving local authorities, the voluntary sector and service users (Welsh Office, 1989). However, an evaluation by the National Audit Office found that it had had only marginal impact, due to a lack of leadership from the Welsh Office, too many targets, inadequate monitoring and difficulty in releasing resources to invest in areas where health gain could be maximised (NAO, 1996b). 'Health gain' and 'health improvement' within a population can mask deepening inequalities between groups. Hence, tracking and addressing social and economic inequalities has to be an explicit task if health inequity is to be tackled.

There was optimism among those working in public health when Labour won the election in 1997. The new Government was looking to a 'third way' between the 'nanny state' that intervenes in people's lives and expects them to take responsibility for looking after themselves and blaming them if they fail. A social exclusion unit was set up in the Prime Minister's office to demonstrate the Government's determination to deal with the rising gap between the rich and poor. Initiatives included Sure Start, neighbourhood renewal, the introduction of a national minimum wage and working family tax credit. An independent inquiry on inequalities in health was set up with Donald Acheson as chair. The report was published in 1998 and made recommendations covering housing, transport and employment (Acheson, 1998).

Saving Lives: Our Healthier Nation was published as the public health strategy for England in 1999. The report accepted that health and wealth go together and that tackling health means addressing economic disadvantage and it placed the emphasis on governments acting on the factors that damage people's health that lie beyond their control (DH, 1999). The strategy, though, was still based on specific diseases that limited the 'ownership' by other agencies and there were no targets around inequalities. Health authorities were expected to develop health implementation plans, working with local authorities and other agencies.

The *NHS Plan*, published in 2000, eclipsed *Saving Lives* and focussed attention once again on how to best organise healthcare. The role of government in reducing inequalities in health by 'joined up government' and tackling vested interests soon shifted back to focus on the individual's role in health promotion and disease prevention. Public health as a specialty continued to decline in comparison with other clinical specialties. In his annual report in 2005 the Chief Medical Officer for Health reported concerns about the striking local and regional differences in expenditure, finding a 20-fold variation in expenditure on health improvement by primary care trusts, much more than could be accounted for by different need. He concluded that unless the situation is addressed, it will have significant implications in future for life expectancy, healthy years of life, demand for NHS services and premature deaths (CMO, 2005).

Pressure groups

The public health agenda is diverse and diffuse making collective action by different pressure groups hard. Three public health groups came together in 1999 to form the UK Public Health Association which campaigns for a boarder public health agenda. Otherwise most health related voluntary sector groups have campaigned to support preventive medicine rather than tackling socioeconomic inequalities. Specific pressure groups have been effective, often those that have a disease or condition-based objective that coincided with other interests. They have often seen public health mainly in terms of more preventive interventions and of inequalities in terms of access to screening or immunisation. There have been successes as a result of pressure groups and the effective use of the media. Action on Smoking and Health (ASH) and Alcohol Concern were single issue groups that took on areas where there were strong vested interest ranged against them – the tobacco and drinks industries. ASH has been particularly successful in achieving controls in smoking in public places. But there was a long history of denial and delay. Changes have been made by retailers who want to present a greener image. Nutritional standards for school meals, the responsibility of the Department of Education and Employment, were abolished in 1980 but were reinstated in 2006 following publicity about the poor nutrition of school meals by celebrity TV chef Jamie Oliver. Public health alerts and campaigns about genetically modified foods have been taken up by the media and raised awareness. However, corporate interests remain powerful, with the political leverage to persuade governments not to adopt health policies inimical to their interests (Baggott, 2007).

Medicalising public health

By the end of the nineteenth century the medical profession had taken over from engineers and social reformers. Victorian sanitary reformers had seen the causes of ill health to be in the environment and poverty, but the discovery of 'germs' led people to see the causes to be not so much in the environment or circumstances of the family but in their knowledge and personal behaviour. The focus of public health changed to approaches which manipulated individual behaviour, mainly women who were mothers, to prevent disease rather than improving the environment. It saw solutions to inequalities in health to lie in interventions such as health education, immunisation and screening – approaches that turn people back into patients, to whom and for whom things are done, rather than expecting them to take action or responsibility for themselves. It is also ineffective in tackling health inequalities. Those most likely to die early are those least likely to present for a diagnosis, respond to screening invitations or keep appointments.

The role demanded of the public is compliance. Some patients' groups have promoted the uptake of screening and immunisation and put pressure on governments to extend screening to other groups. Such campaigns can have the support of powerful professional and commercial interests and this can help their success. Patients' groups may campaign against inequalities for men in cancer screening and against age discrimination in breast cancer screening, but may fail to tackle the wider issues of the evidence for increased interventions or social and economic inequalities and environmental causes of disease. There are costs as well as benefits of interventions and ethical issues in providing health services to apparently healthy people. It has been argued that screening as currently practised is unethical because people are not informed about the risks involved, such as the side-effects of screening tests, incorrect diagnosis and unnecessary treatment. Informed consent that is central now to treatment decisions is not applied to screening and immunisation (Shickle and Chadwick, 1994).

User groups have not generally questioned the benefits of screening but the situation has been different for immunisation. Many immunisation programmes rely on universal coverage. The theory being that if enough people are immunised against a particular disease it will disappear. This benefits poorer families who are more likely to live in inadequate and overcrowded housing. There is, however, a conflict between benefit for the individual and benefit for the community as a whole. By immunising them, healthy children are put at risk of adverse reactions. These are difficult decisions for parents and there is a likelihood that the more information is given to the public, the less likely they are to comply. Parents groups have been effective in undermining public confidence in the MMR (mumps, measles and rubella) vaccine that was introduced in 1988. This has resulted in reduced take-up of the vaccine and significant measles outbreaks. This opposition was not new. There were riots in the nineteenth century against compulsory vaccination against small pox. In 1898 a new Vaccination Act was passed that allowed for exemption for the 'conscientious objector' which resulted in a sharp drop in the number of children being vaccinated (Halvorsen, 2007).

Health education

Health education has traditionally been seen as the way that professionals pass on information to the public who are expected to comply in the same way they do to medical advice when they are ill. Health education began with the public health movement in the nineteenth century. The first emphasis of health education was on cleanliness and hygiene in order to control infectious diseases. Local authorities appointed health visitors to teach mothers about the basic care of infants. Otherwise health promotion rarely got beyond posters exhorting people to wash their hands, brush their teeth or stop smoking. Later the messages became more complex, telling people how to avoid risks to their health and attempting to stop them doing things they may enjoy, such as smoking, eating too much or the wrong foods, unprotected sex, drinking alcohol and using drugs.

In the 1970s and 1980s there was increasing disillusionment with the failures of health education. Traditional health education was not very successful because the messages and methods where chosen by professionals without consulting the people they wanted to influence. Public awareness campaigns continued and still had their uses if only to reassure the public that the government was taking action on drugs, HIV/AIDS, poverty, crime or other issues. But experts accepted they were unlikely to change behaviour.

In the 1970s CHCs were seen to have a role in health promotion because of their links with the community. In *Prevention and Health: Everybody's Business,* CHCs were given a special responsibility for developing the preventive aspects of their work. The Government considered that CHCs could help to transmit the preventive message to the public.[2] Many CHCs undertook health education activities, gave information on health issues to the public, carried out surveys and monitored health education. CHCs justified moving into health promotion because it was something no one else was tackling and it was a way of making the CHC useful to the public and raising its profile with the community. The 'health educators' became a distinctive group within CHCs, seeing a major part of their role as promoting changes in behaviour through health education. CHCs were often at the forefront of good practice in working with community groups and providing information that people wanted. They ran events, often with additional funding from the NHS, to promote the uptake of cervical cancer screening. They ran health fairs and clubs for children to get over messages about healthy lifestyles. A survey in 1985 found that a quarter of CHCs had carried out health education activities for two to 16-year-olds and over 40 percent of CHCs felt that it was important for the CHC to undertake health education (Piette, 1985). There were inevitably criticisms that CHCs should stick to activities where their expertise as community representatives was most appropriate and press for better health promotion services, rather than trying to provide them. The work that CHCs carried out in the early days on health promotion demonstrates both the strength and weaknesses of CHCs. Their remit gave them the flexibility to be creative and fill gaps at a time when health education departments in health authorities were under-resourced and many still saw their role as little more than producing posters. However, it also meant that it was easy for CHCs to lose focus and stray into areas peripheral to their main duties.

Health education techniques have become smarter. Social marketing uses marketing concepts and techniques to achieve specific changes in behaviour for a social or public good. In other words adapting the most effective advertising and marketing techniques to 'sell' health and encourage healthier lifestyles. The National Consumer Council (2006) has suggested that the Department of Health should develop a national social marketing strategy for health. Health education and health promotion, the area where the NHS is most comfortable, was once again in favour, albeit with new clothes – the clothes of health literacy and social marketing.

Self-care and the expertise of experience

In the 1970s and 1980s medical sociologists wrote learned papers about patients' beliefs and understanding. Patients were generally assumed to be in error if they did not agree with professionals or follow their advice. However, there was a trend from the 1980s to talk of lay knowledge and expertise. Patients were no longer wrong in their beliefs, just 'different' from professionals (Prior, 2003). Patients' expertise lay in their experiences which professionals needed to understand in order to identify a course that would lead to a better outcome. The amount of medical knowledge available to health professionals is growing at an exponential rate. For rarer conditions, it is easy for a patient to keep up to date with research on their condition, in a way that is impossible for a general physician (Muir Gray, 2002). Many doctors' immediate response was that better informed patients would take up more of their time (Shaw and Baker, 2004). Others believe that patient engagement is a component of a strategy to keep future health-care spending within manageable limits and that the sustainability of the NHS depends on the effectiveness of efforts to promote more equal relationships between patients and professionals (Coulter, 2006; Muir Gray, 2002).

Promoting self-care was slow to be taken up by the Department of Health. Clive Smee, the Chief Economic Adviser to the Department of Health from 1984–2002, noted that there was resistance because it was thought that self-care might undermine the role of the Department of Health and the NHS and thus lead to a reduction in their funding. There was no formal policy lead in the Department of Health and no vested interests pushing for change, whether professional or patients' groups. There were also concerns that self-care might be interpreted as a policy of the blaming patients or excusing cutbacks (Smee, 2005: 143).

Expert Patient Programme

The Expert Patient Programme was launched in 2001. For the first time promoting self-care became a part of policy based on the belief that self-management programmes can reduce the severity of symptoms and improve patients' confidence and resourcefulness. The programme is a lay-led training programme for people with chronic conditions to help them take more responsibility for the management of their condition and work in partnership with their health and social care providers (DH, 2001a). Participants in the programme are encouraged to become trainers and remain involved.

In *Choosing Health* the Department of Health proposed that NHS health trainers would in future give people in deprived communities help in giving up smoking or healthy eating (DH, 2004a). People would be able to complete an assessment online or on paper and, based on this they would be offered advice, support or signposting to local services. Trainers were to be drawn from local communities so that they understand the day-to-day concerns and experience of people they are supporting.

Many people may benefit from such training programmes. Certainly participants report increased self confidence and self esteem. An internal evaluation by the Department of Health found reductions in the use of health services.[3] However, others have questioned the methodology of the studies and see the interpretation of the results as optimistic (Taylor and Bury, 2007). Others report that such programmes are unlikely to reduce hospital admissions or the use of other healthcare resources (Griffiths et al., 2007). In 2006 management of the Expert Patient Programme was transferred to a not-for-profit community interest company.

A fundamental criticism of such programmes is that they maintain the individual as a patient in the sick role. The Department of Health has estimated that about 60 percent of adults have a chronic illness and are potentially eligible (DH, 2003a). This is higher than other estimates: in the Census 2001, 18.2 percent of people in England and Wales reported that they suffered from a long-term illness or disability that limited daily activities or the work that they could do. By accepting such high levels of chronic disease, the Department of Health is inviting people to become engaged in being ill, which has implications for the wider society. It seems that in more affluent societies we are more likely to perceive ourselves to have poorer health (Sen, 2002). One is reminded that one of the reasons that the Department of Health was slow to take an interest in self-care was because it was felt that it would undermine its role in government (Smee, 2005). It seems that with self-care the Department had found a way to strengthen its position after all.

Choice and the Wanless report

Public health slipped in priority as choice moved up. In 2001 Derek Wanless, a retired banker, was asked by the Treasury to review the long-term funding requirements of healthcare. He based his estimates of costs in the future on the degree to which people become engaged with their own health and so improve the health status of the population. He observed that individuals are responsible for their own and their children's health and it is the aggregate actions of individuals, which ultimately determine demand and how much healthcare in the future will cost (Wanless, 2002). In the Wanless report the Treasury team modelled three scenarios: slow uptake, in which there is no change in the level of public engagement in health and so little or no improvement in health status; solid progress, where people are more engaged, health status improves and people make more appropriate use of health services; and fully engaged, where there is a dramatic improvement in public engagement, coupled with productivity improvements and major improvements in health status due to more effective public health measures. The report concluded that the last scenario, which involved a radical change in professional and public roles, was the most ambitious but offered the best and most cost effective means of matching demand and supply in the long-term.

The Wanless report in 2002 gave a new impetus for public health in the context of individual actions and using 'choice' as a lever for change. It recognised 'systematic failures' that influence the decisions individuals make. These included a lack of information and understanding of the wider social costs of particular behaviours and ingrained social attitudes that are not conducive to individuals pursuing healthy lifestyles (Wanless, 2002). More recently the commercial possibilities of 'well-being' have been noted – with fitness centres, complementary therapies and nutritional supplements providing large new markets.

Addressing lifestyle issues is necessary, but is not enough, and should not be the main focus against a background of inequalities. However, the conclusions of the Wanless report fitted in well with the Government's choice agenda and liberal individualistic approaches which place greater emphasis on people's freedom to pursue activities without interference from the state, providing others are not harmed as a result. People can be given information and then expected to make their choices. The next public health White Paper, *Choosing Health*, in 2004 reflected this vision. The White Paper *Our Health, Our Care, Our Say: A New Direction for Community Services* continued this focus on the support that people need to make choices, but did not address the social determinants of health or the inequalities that are likely to follow more choice (DH, 2006a). The Government now seemed to see itself to have a supportive role to individuals rather than taking responsibility for making the population healthy.

Community development approaches

Community development approaches assume that ensuring healthier communities needs the active consent and involvement of those governed. Communities need to be involved in both identifying the problems and the solutions. Public health professionals tend to be concerned with physical health, such as cancers, immunisation or heart disease, whereas people themselves may give priority to stress, housing or community safety.

Community development encourages informal networks and interagency working. It builds social capital and supports community engagement as well as building up people's self esteem and confidence and overcoming social isolation. Although it is hard to trace a causal relationship between social networks and health, experience indicates that people who feel connected, rather than isolated or excluded, tend to engage more in community activities and to report that they feel healthier as a result (Gilchrist, 2007).

Early community development projects

In the 1970s and 1980s some health promotion professionals moved away from the top-down approach to work with disadvantaged communities to help

Box 7.5   Understanding the impact of inequalities

During this time there was also a better understanding of the impact of health inequalities through the work of Richard Wilkinson and Michael Marmot.

Michael Marmot noted that when whole societies are materially poor, increasing their income makes a difference to their health. But when a society's material needs are met, something different comes into play. The higher in the social hierarchy you are, the better your health. How much control you have over your life is crucial for health and well-being and determines how long you live. Autonomy and the opportunity to participate fully in society are important to health and well-being. Marmot first observed this in a long-term study of the health of Whitehall civil servants. To the surprise of the researchers it was not the high powered mandarins who suffered from stress, but those lower down the hierarchy. Marmot calls this the 'status syndrome'. The phenomenon has been noted in many rich countries and even in primates. Therefore, he concludes the key issue for public policy in wealthy countries is to understand what it is about the way we live that effects our health.

Richard Wilkinson's research on international comparisons of inequalities demonstrated the socially corrosive effects of inequality and the psychosocial impact of class stratification. People living in societies with great distance between the richest and the poorest feel more hostility, are less likely to become involved in community life and much less likely to trust each other. They are likely to have higher rates of violent crime and homicide. Furthermore, there is a tendency for societies with bigger inequalities to show more discrimination against vulnerable groups, such as women, religious or ethnic minorities. In unequal societies with a big gap between rich and poor, everybody's health and length of life is affected, the rich as well as the poor. Societies with large inequalities have lower levels of 'social capital'. The idea of social capital recognises that social networks are a valuable asset which enables people to build communities, to commit themselves to each other, and knits the social fabric together.

Sources: Marmot, 2004; Wilkinson, 2005.

them look for ways to improve their health. Community development aims to enable people to solve problems and meet their needs as they see them. Unlike traditional health education, community development approaches do not expect individuals to help themselves (and blame them if they fail), but expect communities to help improve health and well-being both directly and indirectly by acting collectively on the environmental causes of disease.

Community involvement had been 'discovered' as a way to tackle deprivation and inequalities in the 1960s. The Seebohm Report on social services in 1968 emphasised community-based social services. Community schools were developed in targeted areas with more involvement of parents and local communities. Community development projects were set up to see if public participation could revitalise disadvantaged areas (see Box 7.5). CHCs had their roots in these ideas. Some CHCs took up environmental issues, including housing, pesticides and the potential hazards of people living with nuclear installations, where there were above the national rates of childhood leukemia. North Devon CHC drew attention to the problems of families living near a chemical plan near Falkirk where there were cases of deformed and sick cattle and cases of babies born with severe eye defects. Durham CHC took up health problems following crop spraying.[4]

Health for All

While responsibility and expertise in public health lay with the NHS, local authorities took up the task of working with disadvantaged communities, drawing their inspiration from international rather than national strategies. The Declaration of Alma Ata in 1978 of Health for All by the Year 2000 was an inspirational rallying cry. Participation was deeply embedded in Health for All, from which came initiatives such as Healthy Cities, where the city was the focal point for a range of health promotion interventions. A key part of the definition and objectives of a 'healthy city' was the involvement of citizens and tackling inequalities. Belfast, Glasgow, Liverpool and the London Borough of Camden were established as 'healthy cities' in the UK. Soon Health for All became a movement and other local authorities adopted strategies tried out by the 'healthy cities'. It coincided with increasing concerns in inner city authorities about the health of their communities. However, the values and strategies did not fit in with national policies and community health strategies did not become part of the mainstream NHS.

Agenda 21

Local authorities also took the lead in developing strategies for Agenda 21 (an Agenda for the twenty-first century). This was agreed by 180 world leaders at the United Nations Earth Summit in Rio de Janeiro in 1992. Agenda 21 is an action plan for achieving sustainable development at national, regional and local levels. Some local authorities took up Agenda 21 with enthusiasm as a way of integrating social, environmental and economic aspects of sustainable development and improving the environment in which people live and work. One of the more successful aspects of Agenda 21 was the experimentation with new approaches to participation. In 2000 community strategies, which have a striking similarity to local Agenda 21 strategies, were made a statutory duty for all local authorities. Agenda 21 strategies were marginal institutionally; community strategies are potentially more effective (Lucas et al., 2001).

Tackling social exclusion

At the start of the Labour Government in 1997 there was some enthusiasm for community development approaches to tackle inequalities and social exclusion. Healthy living centres were launched in 1997 which recognised the value of working with disadvantaged communities on their own terms (DH, 1998b). Three hundred and forty-nine healthy living centres were funded through the Big Lottery for five years. Health authorities were given a greater role in public health: they were expected to develop health implementation plans, working with local authorities and other agencies and were given additional funds to target disadvantaged areas with Health Action Zones.

Commissioning provides opportunities for primary care trusts to respond to the needs of the population and invest in health gain. Health impact assessment is a method by which the impact of a policy or programme on the health of local people is assessed in order to achieve better and more robust decisions. Public involvement in health impact assessment provides important evidence because understanding the complex responses people have to social and economic structures improves the understanding of what is possible. People may interpret risk in a different way from professionals. Public involvement in health impact assessment can help recast the relationships between communities and decision-makers in a more democratic way and build social capital (Elliott et al., 2004).

In practice needs assessments have tended to focus on a narrow view of health gain and on the needs of local people for clinical services and remain a professional rather than participative activities. Primary care trusts are expected to base their commissioning on the evidence of effectiveness of interventions, which inevitably gives a bias towards treatment and care since it is easier to demonstrate the effectiveness of treatment than of public health interventions. For public health interventions, randomised controlled trials do not work since the variables are hard and often impossible to control. There may be tensions for commissioners where government targets are set based on national priorities and a medicalised view of inequalities and ill health.

While public health policies were focussing on the individual, there were other national policies which, if developed, would give priority to healthy public policies Industrial society is damaging because of its tendency to create unhealthy lifestyles and working patterns as well as producing socioeconomic inequalities that undermine health. The impact of inequalities on all aspects of society is increasingly better understood (Box 7.4). Policies that impact health include economic sustainability, 'green' issues, well-being and local decision-making. The environmental lobby emphasises the complex causes of illness arising from environment in which people live, in particular, problems with food manufacturing and diseases linked to pollution. They have adopted an ecological model of health which places an emphasis on the many sources of illness in the environment. Health problems, such as Bovine Spongiform Encephalitis (BSE) and bird flu, obesity, pollution and the widening health gap between the rich and poor are viewed as a result of our exploitation of the environment. A government report on obesity identified how much the environment was implicated in growing levels of obesity (Foresight, 2007). It concluded that tackling obesity is similar to tackling climate change. Both need whole societal change with cross-government action and long-term commitment. Many climate change goals will also help to prevent obesity, such as measures to reduce traffic congestion, increase cycling or design sustainable communities. There would also be synergies with other policy goals, such as increasing social inclusion and narrowing health inequalities since obesity's impact is greatest on the poorest (see Box 7.2). It is perhaps in this way that public pressure will be put on governments to tackle the environmental causes of diseases, such as breast cancer and obesity.

Conclusions

From *Health is Everybody's Business* in 1976 to the Wanless report in 2002, governments have looked at policies that could help achieve healthier people and reduce the increases in the costs of providing healthcare. After over 30 years of national public health strategies, the NHS remains essentially a sickness service. The Department of Health and the NHS always seems to return to interventions for specific diseases and targeting communities to increase their access to healthcare and preventive medicine. There has been a long-term failure to develop healthy public policies (Scott-Samuel and Wills, 2007).

There remain many barriers to a major shift in the balance of resources or activities towards promoting public health. A major barrier is the confused thinking in national health policy about tackling inequalities and passing responsibility to individuals. Is it up to citizens to eat and drink appropriately, or should the state provide good advice or should companies sell healthier food? In line with other policies in healthcare there is a trend to put risks and responsibilities on the individual for their own health. This emphasis on individual responsibility for one's own health is likely to form an increasingly important part of patient and public involvement in the future. However, this can increase inequalities in health since for some people adopting a healthier lifestyle will be difficult, whether because of genetic differences, lack of education, poverty, deep-seated cultural traditions, or other factors that make it hard for them. Failure to make healthy choices, may lead to further disadvantage.

However, even with the best will in the world, action on public health was outside the Department of Health's powers, if not its remit. The Department of Health's lead responsibility for public health has perpetuated a persistent bias towards providing a sickness service rather than looking at wider issues of prevention. The Department of Health has a wider remit than the English NHS, but this has become less important. A senior civil servant said in 2006: '*The Department of Health [DH] is the best example where the traditional mandarin is a species threatened with extinction. The danger here is that the DH runs the risk of almost perfect producer capture*' (Lodge and Rogers, 2006: 31). It has increasingly focussed on the English NHS and not the wider determinants of health, and compares unfavourably with the other UK countries. Greer and Jarman (2007) argue that it needs to be rebalanced in order to redevelop its potential role as a UK Department of Health rather than the English NHS.

Reducing ill health requires tackling inequalities in health and this requires broader interagency action to address the wider problems of society, including low self esteem, stress, crime and violence as well as poverty and housing. In spite of the evidence of its failures, the NHS is still expected to take the lead in public health. Public health faces three major challenges, which cannot be resolved by individuals or by the NHS. These are: chronic and long-term conditions, including mental illness and obesity; health improvement and tackling health inequalities; and redefining the role of the hospital in health services so that it no longer dominates both policy and use of resources (Hunter, 2004). There are barriers to co-operation between primary care trusts and local authorities, which may be easier with largely coterminous boundaries between primary care trusts and local authorities introduced in 2006, but this will not overcome the basic differences in philosophy and approach. With this in mind, it may be that the future of public health will lie with local authorities once again. Local authorities have lacked legitimacy in public health, but this may be changing with overview and scrutiny committees and their new role as community leaders. Promoting the health of disadvantaged communities is a major part of the initiatives to engage citizens and rebuild democracy which are discussed in Chapter 10.

Past Imperfect...
Abolishing CHCs

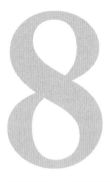

'*Present imperfect but better than future ghastly... The government seems to have decided to abolish CHCs in a fit of pique – perhaps over the persistent objections to the Public Finance Initiative, perhaps in revenge for the yearly embarrassment inflicted by Casualty Watch, perhaps over some personality clash. It should rethink. If CHCs did not exist, we probably would want to invent them. Perhaps not in their present form, perhaps with wholly different funding arrangements. But the NHS needs something like them and the more effective the better*'.

Editorial, *Health Service Journal*, 7 September 2000, p. 19.

Overview

This chapter outlines the events that led up to the abolition of CHCs and the impact of campaigns against abolition.

- CHCs wanted reform but opposed abolition.
- They campaigned to make the new forums more like CHCs with significant success, but in doing so antagonised the government.
- Most of the amendments and commitments they achieved were not implemented and there was no transition for staff or members to the new patients' forums.

This chapter is based on interviews with key participants in these events as part of a research study.

Introduction

In 1997 CHCs had reason to be optimistic – the Labour Party had been sympathetic to them in government and in opposition. After 1997 there was a new interest in patient and public involvement from government. In spite of the political rhetoric, little priority had been given to work on patient involvement before 1997. The unit within the Department of Health with policy responsibility was lightly staffed, staff turnover was quite rapid and recognition and support from senior management were limited (Smee, 2005: 143). New agencies, such as the Commission for Health Improvement, the National Patient Safety Agency (NPSA) and the National Institute for Clinical Excellence (NICE) sought to involve patients and carers. In 2002 patient and public involvement in England got its own 'tsar' and Harry Cayton became national director of the patient experience and public involvement. The National Primary Care Development Programme developed its competency framework for engagement and strategic health authorities implemented performance management frameworks for patient and public involvement.

There were signs of difficulties ahead for CHCs. A warning had been issued by an expert group commissioned by the NHS Executive, the Institute of Health Service Management and the NHS Confederation to make recommendations about public participation in the NHS. It suggested that CHCs should have a more focussed role and become 'professional scrutineers' with a remit for reviewing the contribution of health and local authority services, auditing policies of public authorities to assess their impact and inspecting health services and facilities (Bridge Consultancy, 1998). It suggested that CHCs could report to the Commission for Health Improvement, responsible for regulating standards in health service nationally. Though the report seemed to reflect what many CHCs were saying, the *Health Service Journal*, the voice of NHS managers, saw it as 'damning' and an important landmark: the first time the NHS Executive had explicitly acknowledged that CHCs were not fulfilling their role. It concluded that the findings had come '*amid rumours of ministers' intense dissatisfaction with CHCs' performance and internal turmoil at the Association of CHCs for England and Wales, are bound to ignite controversy*'.[1]

Frank Dobson, the Secretary of State, noted that the Government would need to look at where CHCs would fit into the 'new NHS' at the ACHCEW AGM in 1998. But he added: '*For the time being, keep on doing what you are already doing, but do it a bit better as well*'.[2] There were clearly going to be changes in England and CHCs had been told that they needed to prove themselves.

While in England CHCs were abolished, in Wales they were reformed. In Scotland and Northern Ireland new arrangements were developed, based on different models of user involvement (see Chapter 10).

The calm before the storm

CHCs themselves were finally united behind the need for change and they were expecting the long awaited reforms. Unfortunately, the movement was not in a healthy state to meet this challenge or demonstrate its capacity to develop. Problems within ACHCEW that had been simmering for many years came to the fore. There had been longstanding conflicts about the most appropriate role for a CHC and the respective roles of members and staff. The ACHCEW office, while respected for the quality of its work, was not seen as CHC-friendly. Apart from the first Director, no member of staff had been appointed who had worked in a CHC. Toby Harris was facing difficulties in his relationships with some CHCs and this came to a head in 1998. With the Chair's agreement, he had accepted a non-executive directorship of the London ambulance service trust which some CHCs saw as a conflict of interest. He had left in July 1998, before becoming Lord Harris of Haringey, against a *'dismal backdrop of boardroom division and festering acrimony between the organisation's leadership and a sizable chunk of its membership'*.[3] In his farewell speech to the AGM he observed that CHCs would disappear into a footnote of NHS history *'and some people will be delighted to dance on the grave'* if they did not grasp the opportunities for modernisation now.[4] After he had left the rebellion continued over the appointment of his replacement. Some CHC staff thought this was an opportunity to evaluate the role of Director and involve CHCs more in the appointment.[5]

Donna Covey became Director in 1998 and energetically set out to get CHCs on the map. She set up an All-Party Parliamentary Group on CHCs, which in 1999 had 240 MPs in membership, many of whom had been CHC members. She also set up an independent commission with Will Hutton, then Editor-in-Chief of the Observer, as the chair. The resulting report looked at ways of strengthening and reforming CHCs in the context of accountability in the NHS (Hutton, 2000).

But the problems did not go away. Membership of ACHCEW was declining and only 132 out of 200 CHCs attended the AGM in July 2000. At this AGM for the first time in its history one of the vice chairs stood against the chair for election and won by 62 votes to 60. Sadly this was not fought on policy, principles, strategy or the future of CHCs but on personalities – causing an old fashioned split on lines of gender, social class, and the North, South and London divides. This split further destabilised ACHCEW and affected its credibility in the outside world.

The timing could not have been worse. There were signs that the Government was already looking elsewhere for answers. The Government wanted to engage directly with the public. What the Government called *'the biggest ever Listening Exercise'* was launched on the 9 May 2000. This included a 'Census Day' for the NHS on 31 May to gather as many views as possible from the public, patients and staff. Twelve million leaflets asking for the public to feedback their views were made available in every hospital, GP surgery as well as supermarkets and high street chemists. A dedicated internet website was set up for people to express their views and two public meetings held in Leeds and London of 100 people.[6] This was an impressive exercise, but given that the *NHS Plan* was to be published in July, it is doubtful that any results could be taken into account.

Specialist advisory groups, modernisation action teams, were set up with members from the professions, unions and voluntary organisations to advise ministers, including one on patient care (empowerment). Key people from the voluntary sector became influential in national policy as part of the modernisation action teams at this time. Harry Cayton from the Alzheimer's Society, David Harker from Citizens Advice, Melinda Letts from the Long-term Medical Conditions Alliance, Cliff Prior from Rethink and Paul Streets from

Diabetes UK. They provided a different and more patient/consumerist focus from CHCs. A civil servant noted: '*They had been very influential in describing different models of engagement and provided a powerful new perspective. In the past the Department had not engaged in this way with the voluntary sector. This was a contrast to ACHCEW*' (Hogg, 2006b). Though ACHCEW was excluded from this advisory group, the question of abolition was apparently not raised or discussed; apparently it recommended the strengthening of CHCs.[7,8]

The NHS Plan

However, discussions were going on behind the scenes at a senior level in Whitehall about abolishing CHCs. In 1998 there had been rumours that the Prime Minister's office in Downing Street was thinking of replacing CHCs with patient representatives in each hospital. There were rumours that Alan Millburn, Secretary of State, personally did not support CHCs. Gisela Stuart, as Minister, cancelled a planned speech at the 2000 ACHCEW conference because of 'Whitehall commitments'.[9] A civil servant also due to speak at the conference had been told that he should not attend. According to Gisela Stuart the final decision was only made after the ACHCEW AGM. She did not want to abolish them. She felt that CHCs had been a good model that had worked well in the past, but some had become inward-looking political cliques. But the problem remained of how reform might be implemented. Asking ACHCEW to take over the budget and reform of CHCs was considered, but it was concluded that it did not have the leadership or capacity to do this. She did not feel that it was appropriate for the Department of Health to reform or manage what had to be local bodies. Having come to this conclusion, there was no option but to abolish CHCs and start again. After a brainstorming session with her advisers after the ACHCEW AGM, Chapter 10 of the *NHS Plan* was written (Hogg, 2006c).

On 27 July 2000 the *NHS Plan* was published. The intention was to '*give the people of Britain a health service designed around the patient*' (DH, 2000: 10). The Government stated the intention was to move away from '*an outdated system of patients being on the outside*'. It was a new model where the '*voices of patients, and their carers and the public are heard throughout every level of the service, acting as a powerful lever for change and improvement*' (DH, 2001b: 2). Chapter 10 of the *NHS Plan* proposed a range of new arrangements to support patient and public involvement (see Box 8.1). The *Plan* concluded: '*these are far reaching and fundamental reforms which will bring patients and citizens into decision-making at every level...... As a result community health councils will be abolished*' (DH, 2000: 10.25). The Plan was endorsed in its preface by 25 representatives from the professions, Royal Colleges, trade unions and the voluntary sector. As the draft plan did not include reference to the abolition of CHCs and the intention was not leaked, many of the signatories were not aware at the time that they were also endorsing the abolition of CHCs.

Box 8.1   Chapter 10 of the NHS Plan

Proposals in the plan covered:

The introduction of a **patient advocacy and liaison service (PALS)** in every trust to take on the role, which community health councils currently filled, of supporting patients with particular problems and steering them towards the complaints process.

Patients' forums were to be established in every NHS and primary care trust to provide direct input from patients into how local NHS services were to be run. *'For the first time patients will have a direct representation on every trust board – elected by the patients' forum. The patients' forum will have half of its members drawn from local patients' groups and voluntary organisations. The other half of the forum members will be randomly drawn from respondents to the trust's annual patient survey. The forum will be supported by the new patient advocacy and liaison service, and will have the right to in visit and inspect any aspect of the trust's care at any time'* (DH, 2000: 10.25).

Citizens would also be represented. Each health authority would have an independent local advisory forum chosen from residents in the area to provide a sounding board for determining health priorities and policies. There would also be increased lay membership on professional regulatory bodies, and other national statutory agencies. This looked remarkably like the advisory panels proposed by the Labour Government in 1970 that predated the design of CHCs.

Local government was to be given the power to scrutinise the NHS, taking over the scrutiny function of CHCs and their right of appeal to the Secretary of State.

Reactions to the Plan

The Labour Government was prepared to take on CHCs, a challenge which other governments since 1980 had ducked. Ministers knew it would be controversial, but felt it would be worth it. The draft *NHS Plan* that had been circulated had not included any reference to the abolition of CHCs. This was to avoid any leaks. Announcing abolition in the *NHS Plan*, which was likely to receive a positive welcome overall, would, it was hoped, reduce the political fallout from the abolition of CHCs.

Shock and disbelief met the announcement. CHCs and others who had dealings with CHCs had not foreseen this. Though there had been rumours that Ministers wanted to abolish CHCs, these were discounted because of the support that CHCs had received at local level. A draft policy consultation document produced by the Labour Party, *Partnership in Power*, had been lukewarm about CHCs, but after two years of consultation with the grass roots the final document, endorsed by the Labour Party Conference in 1999, was more positive. The abolition of CHCs did not reflect what the public said they had wanted in the 'Listening Exercise' or the recommendations of the modernisation action team.

The Director of ACHCEW was informed just before the announcement was made by the Prime Minister in the Commons. Even civil servants were taken by surprise. One commented: 'We *had been working on the reform of CHCs. The first I heard about abolition was when the NHS Plan was published.... Arguments for abolition were not proffered by civil servants or the modernisation action team. That part was written by the Secretary of State... We (civil servants) did not have much say... Special advisers and the private sector were replacing civil servants at the top level'* (Walsh, 2002: 65).

There were many rumours about the 'real' reason for the decision, mainly revolving around Alan Milburn. Some thought it was because he had a bad relationship with his constituency CHC which was not especially true (Gerrard, 2006). There was also a belief that the decision to abolish CHCs had been made at the last minute over a weekend and personally added to the draft plan either by Alan Milburn or his adviser on a laptop. It was said that the Minister responsible, Gisela Stuart, opposed the plan and had been pre-sented with a fait accompli on 19 July by the Secretary of State.[10] Such rumours were also apparently not true.

These were persistent stories, more acceptable than reality. In fact among Ministers there was no support for keeping CHCs or for reform. CHCs and their local intelligence were useful for a party in opposition, but potentially damaging for a party in government. CHCs were seen by Ministers as the last bastion of old Labour and a block to progress. CHCs were not reticent in criticising government policies. For many years ACHCEW had orchestrated CasualtyWatch where CHC members visited and monitored their local A&E departments over the same 24-hour period and the subsequent report always received wide press coverage. It tended to illustrate the discrepancy between national spin and realities on the ground. These campaigns had been very successful initially and achieved targets around A&E waiting times, though some within ACHCEW felt at the time it was unwise to repeat it every year. Greer (2004a) points out that CHCs had led opposition to PFI schemes in many areas and might have been perceived as obstructing the government's strategy for financing new buildings. It had not helped the CHC movement that two Ministers, Gisela Stuart and Philip Hunt, had both run into diffi-culties with one of the CHCs in Birmingham and their campaign against the Public Finance Initiative. Ministers found they were funding an organisation to attack them, which did not make sense.

The extent and strength of the support for CHCs was woefully under-estimated. Many political activists were involved in CHCs and so members had contacts they could use. There were two views among CHCs about how they should respond: one view was to oppose the plans outright and the other to negotiate and try to construct something similar to CHCs. There was, though, agreement that CHCs had to campaign against the proposals to gain a better bargaining position. Once it had recovered from the shock, ACHCEW began mobilising the campaign. The Director of ACHCEW had a trade union background and the skills and experience to develop a concerted political cam-paign: she felt that, as a trade body, ACHCEW had to oppose the abolition of CHCs (Hogg, 2006d). The announcement brought CHCs together as never before. CHCs who had previously not been members of ACHCEW joined up – almost for the first time in its history all CHCs were in membership. Before

July 2000 not all CHCs had e-mail addresses, but by September they all did.

Things did not go well for the appeasers and moderates among CHCs. Ministers felt that they had made their decision and there was nothing to negotiate. After the announcement Ministers refused to meet ACHCEW. In frustration ACHCEW threatened to take a judicial review on the grounds of lack of consultation. When ACHCEW asked the Department of Health to fund this legal action, Alan Milburn, not surprisingly, refused and wrote that he had been advised that the suggestion that the '*courts would intervene to restrain the introduction of primary legislation, for the consideration of Parliament, is without precedent and contrary to basic constitutional principles*'.[11] In the end the judicial review was not pursued. But ACHCEW did achieve one concession – it would survive as long as CHCs did. Earlier the Government had hoped to close ACHCEW before CHCs by withdrawing funding.

Ministers do not like surprises or to be backed into a corner. ACHCEW eventually got a meeting with the Minister, but there seemed to be no point of understanding between them. ACHCEW's Director said '*We never understood why Ministers acted the way they did and why they handled the whole matter so badly, not just the abolition, but afterwards. We had been left in uncertainty.... Ministers just could not understand why we were angry... If they had gone for negotiation, there would have been no great fight. Most CHCs are not radical and would have agreed with plans, as long as there was a national body. Because of the way ministers behaved CHCs got angrier and angrier as time went on*' (Hogg, 2006d). Further anger was caused when the Prime Minister, Tony Blair, claimed in answer to a parliamentary question to Conservative MP Stephen O'Brien in November that he was '*aware that there is bitter opposition, which is why the proposals are being consulted on*' and would be reported '*back to the House in due course on the consultation*'.[12] The Prime Minister later retracted this in a three page letter to the MP.[13]

However, if CHCs were more united than ever before, ACHCEW was not. There were divisions within ACHCEW's management. There were clashes over governance and its relationship with regional associations and between members of the committee and the chair. London CHCs had a well established association, London Health Link. The Chair of London Health Link was well connected and talked to civil servants and briefed members of the House of Lords on its own account. She persuaded the Department of Health to meet all regional associations to seek their views. To some in ACHCEW this was seen as undermining its position. There was also an acrimonious split between ACHCEW and the Society of CHC Staff who saw co-operation as the best way to get a transition deal for staff.[14] The Society did not represent all CHC staff and some staff supported ACHCEW's campaign. However, it was a division that the Department of Health could and did exploit in the debates about the abolition.[15] In spite of the internal tensions, which were perhaps inevitable in the circumstances, ACHCEW managed to maintain a united front throughout.

The first Act

The Health and Social Care Bill was published and ACHCEW turned its attention to campaigning, which had always been one of its strengths. The events are summarised in Box 8.2. ACHCEW wanted amendments to the legislation to replicate CHCs as far as they could. In this they were remarkably successful, achieving many concessions in the Bill. Critics were concerned that the 572 forums replacing 180 CHCs would not be independent and the views of patients and public would be fragmented and their activities unco-ordinated. As a concession, it was agreed to establish additional bodies known as patients' councils that would co-ordinate patients' forums within a health authority area and pursue issues affecting more than one trust or PCT. CHCs also argued against the proposed advisory panel for health authorities: they would not be independent and would have no powers. CHCs and advocacy groups argued that the proposed patient advocacy and liaison services

---

Box 8.2   Summary of events

July 2000 – NHS Plan announces the abolition of CHCs.

December 2000 – Health and Social Care Bill presented to Parliament.

February 2001 – scoping study commissioned by Department of Health on whether the should be a national body to replace ACHCEW.

May 2001 – Health and Social Care Act 2001 passed which put in place for arrangements for overview and scrutiny committees, independent complaints advocacy. Section 12 gave NHS bodies the duty to consult.

June 2001 – General election, Hazel Blears replaces Gisela Stuart as Minister responsible for patient and public involvement.

September 2001 – 'Listening exercise' – six week consultation on new proposals.

November 2001 – Response to the 'Listening Exercise' and NHS and Healthcare Professions Bill published.

February 2002 – Transition Advisory Board holds first meeting.

May 2002 – NHS and Healthcare Professions Act passed.

July 2002 – David Lammy replaces Hazel Blears as minister responsible for patient and public involvement.

July 2002 – Chair Designate of the Commission for Patient and Public Involvement in Health appointed.

September 2002 – Department of Health asks strategic health authorities to set up change action teams to look at how the new forums might be configured in their area.

December 2002 – Transition Advisory Board is disbanded.

January 2003 – Commission for Patient and Public Involvement in Health starts formal work.

July 2003 – ACHCEW moves to wind up at a special general meeting.

November 2003 – CHCs are abolished.

December 2003 – Patients' forums start work.

(PALS) could not provide support for complainants, which needed to be independent of the body about which the complaint was made. As a result an amendment was accepted that required the Secretary of State to ensure that independent advocacy was provided to complainants and 'advice' replaced 'advocacy' in the PALS' title.

Another important concession was the creation of a new national statutory body to replace ACHCEW. Voluntary organisations were increasingly interested in how they could influence national policy (Baggott et al., 2005). They realised that by working together they could have a stronger voice. At this time some voluntary organisations felt that the Government was trying to 'divide and rule' them. Some organisations were perceived to have a special relationship with government – and they were represented on national working groups to the exclusion of other user voices (Hogg et al., 2006). The interest among the voluntary sector coincided with arguments that the new system of patient and public involvement required a national body to ensure coherence and consistency, to monitor standards and provide support for local bodies. The Department of Health commissioned a scoping study from three voluntary organisations (the Patients Forum, Consumers Association and the Long-term Medical Conditions Alliance) while the legislation was going through Parliament. The consultation was carried out in six weeks in order to make sure that the main findings would be available to ministers before it was too late to introduce any additions into legislation. Voluntary organisations, CHCs, professional bodies and other stakeholders were consulted.

There was general support for a publicly-funded national body with rights to information and to be consulted. Most wanted a national body with members and regional networks that could support local involvement and communicate with the national organisation which would include both the voluntary sector and those involved in the new statutory arrangements. CHCs were particularly eager and saw the new body as a way of ensuring that the new arrangements, which they saw as flawed, could develop and have a national profile. The voluntary sector and others were more sceptical, questioning whether a creation of government could be representative of wider patient or public views (Hogg and Graham, 2001). The Government included proposals for a national body in the Bill. This was to be a very different animal from ACHCEW. The main attraction was the possibility of ensuring that the new forums had performance standards and would avoid the variability of CHCs.

An election had been expected in May 2001 but was delayed until June because of an outbreak of foot and mouth disease. The House of Lords had passed amendments the Government could not accept. With an election only weeks away the Government could either withdraw the sections about CHCs or hold up a major piece of legislation and use the Parliament Act to overrule the House of Lord's veto. Once an election is called there are a few days to clear all legislation. This was an opportunity to do a deal and ACHCEW was in a strong negotiating position. An amendment was agreed between the Government and the Liberal Democrats in the House of Lords. Though this got rid of CHCs, they would be replaced by patients' councils which seemed to be recreating CHCs under a new name. Negotiations on the transition of staff and members would follow. However, the Liberal Democrats were not prepared to sign up unless ACHCEW agreed in writing. MPs on the campaign trail did not want to face electors accusing them of abolishing CHCs. ACHCEW was in an impossible situation. The ACHCEW Director, though she agreed that this was the best that they were likely to get, was not willing or able to put in writing her support for the abolition. She reported: '*There was a misunderstanding about my role as director. They did not understand that I work under the direction of the Chair and the Standing Committee and could not make decisions just like that*' (Hogg, 2006d).

So in the end the clauses relating to CHCs were removed in order to get the Bill through. ACHCEW was blamed by politicians for this failure and the misunderstandings continued. The chair of a regional association expressed the view of many CHCs: '*It was a difficult decision to make but ACHCEW did not assess what the impact would be if they refused a deal and made the government and two political parties look stupid just before an election*' (Hogg, 2006e). The proposal for patients' councils, which had given the best opportunity for continuity with CHCs, did not get government support in the second Bill.

CHCs were losing sympathy within the NHS. ACHCEW was a statutory body but was seen to be behaving like a pressure group. This tended to confirm prejudices among NHS managers that CHCs were left of centre and did not behave in a way that statutory bodies should.

The Listening Exercise

CHCs had a reprieve, but the legislation had been passed that would make them redundant. The framework for independent complaints advocacy (ICAS), patients' advice and liaison services (PALS), and overview and scrutiny committees (OSCs) was already in place, each taking over some of the activities of CHCs. The Health and Social Care Act 2001 also included a duty on health bodies a duty to consult (Section 11) for England and Wales.

However, after the election there seemed to be a new sympathy for CHCs. Hazel Blears was appointed to replace Gisela Stuart as the Minister responsible for taking the legislation through Parliament. She had been the chair of Salford and District CHC and the Secretary to the All-Party Parliamentary Group on CHCs. She admitted that the Government had 'got it wrong' when it moved to axe CHCs.[16] A six week consultation exercise was undertaken in the autumn of 2001 and Hazel Blears attended regional consultation events. This did not, however, consult on whether or not to abolish CHCs, just the arrangements that would follow their abolition. The resulting discussion document promised: '*We will not only ensure that everything CHCs currently do will be picked up in the new arrangements, but that patient and citizen involvement will be strengthened and, as a result, will become part of day-to-day NHS activity*' (DH, 2001c: 1.6).

The response to the consultation was published in the November (DH, 2001d). CHCs had achieved much of what they wanted, in particular a new

---

Box 8.3   Proposals following the Listening Exercise

1. Statutory patients' forums would be established, attached to all trusts.
   - PCT forums would have a wider remit and were able to link in with wider health debates.
   - Patients' forum members would have the right to elect a member as a non-executive director to the trust board.
2. A national statutory body, the Commission for Public and Patient Involvement in Health would be set up to oversee the new arrangements, appoint members, set standards, provide training for patients' forums and commission ICAS. A key role for the new Commission was be to ensure that the new arrangements were evaluated and could adapt and be responsive to changes in the NHS.
   - The membership of the Commission was to be drawn mainly from people at local level with relevant expertise, with nominations from forums and the Commission's local networks. Membership would also consist of a national stakeholder group.
   - The Commission's responsibilities were widened to include representing the interests of patients and the public in the delivery of NHS services. Its findings were to be used by the Health Select Committee and by Parliament nationally to hold the Department of Health to account.
   - The Commission was also give a wider role in building the capacity within communities for engagement and co-ordinating activities over strategic health authority areas with staffed local networks with an accessible base.
3. In the discussion document it had been proposed to set up separate statutory bodies called Voice at strategic health authority level with specialist staff to strengthen and facilitate the public voice. There were concerns about the independence and accountability of the professional staff and it was decided that the Commission would employ staff who would be accountability to a national lay group.

Source: DH, 2001b: 3.56.

---

independent statutory body with more power and status than ACHCEW had. There was talk of transition from the old to the new. Short of ensuring their own survival CHCs and their allies had achieved a lot. Thinking in the Department of Health had changed radically (see Box 8.3).

The second Act

After this interlude, the battle commenced again in November 2001 with the NHS and Healthcare Professions Bill. Over the summer the Director of ACHCEW had felt that focussing on transition would be the best way to ensure that CHC staff and members got the best deal out of the new arrangements. A transition advisory board had been proposed in the report of the Listening Exercise and was a key part of the strategy to appease opposition to the new Bill as it went through Parliament. The Secretary of State reported that it had already been set up and meeting in November 2001 in the second reading of the Bill, though it was not set up till two months later.

The ACHCEW Director proposed that the board should be supported by ACHCEW with funding from the Department of Health. This had been agreed verbally with the Department of Health before she moved to a new job in November 2001 and was replaced by Peter Walsh, previously the Chief Officer of Croydon CHC. However, some honorary officers and the new director were not happy with this arrangement. They felt that it would inhibit their ability to campaign about the legislation. Officials in the Department of Health also seemed to go cool on the proposal and proposed instead an independent board.

ACHCEW, released from the need to co-operate in its own demise, continued to brief MPs and members of the House of Lords and campaign for the changes it wanted. As before it fought a vigorous and successful campaign, causing maximum embarrassment for the Government. Through the opposition spokesmen in the House of Lords, Earl Howe and Lord Clement Jones, an amendment to have patients' councils was passed against the Government and was perhaps the greatest moment of ACHCEW's campaign. While there was still support for CHCs and anger for the way they were being treated, generally the voluntary sector felt that it was time to move on. Few, however, were prepared overtly to support the Government and abolition. During the debate in the House of Lords in April 2002, the Chair of the Long-term Medical Conditions Alliance wrote to every member of the House of Lords urging them to reject the proposed amendments.[17] However, the impact backfired since the envelope of her letter was identical – with an identical label – to an envelope containing a letter from the Minister also urging rejection of the amendment. Both letters, it seemed, had been dispatched centrally by the Department of Health.

The amendment to set up patients' councils was overturned in the Commons but the Government made several concessions to the CHC lobby. It was agreed that the PCT patients' forums would have additional responsibilities to promote, encourage and support public involvement in health; provide advice to the NHS and other bodies on public involvement; and to represent public views on matters affecting their health, widening their remit to areas outside NHS services. Another concession achieved was that forums would have their own staff directly accountable to them and hold their own budgets, in the same way that CHCs had. This was seen a way of transferring CHC staff to forums.

The model for forums had changed to make them member-led organisations, with staff in a supportive rather than proactive role. Ministers wanted the new forums to be member-led and get away from the situation in some CHCs where staff were seen as the public face and undertook most of the work. Each forum was required to have a majority of either current or ex-patients and at least one representative of a patient or carers organisation. In the case of PCT forums, local residents were to make up a majority of the members and they had to include at least one person from a body representing residents in matters of their health, as well as at least one representative from each of the trust forums in their area. There was a desire to recruit new people not previously involved and get away from people who were pejoratively referred to as the 'usual suspects' – that is people who were already involved in CHCs or voluntary organisations.

In order to get the legislation through, Parliament was promised that PCT forums would be 'one-stop shops' in the way that CHCs had been. PCT patients' forums were given the function of assisting patients, families and carers in prescribed circumstances as well as responsibility for providing or commissioning ICAS. Neither of these concessions was implemented.

The Act set up a new independent statutory body, Commission for Patient and Public Involvement in Health (CPPIH). It was given a wide range of functions, including:

- The responsibility for promoting patient and public involvement in the NHS;
- The recruitment and appointment of members of patients' forums;
- The employment of staff to support forums; and
- Setting standards for, and performance management of, forums and ICAS.

It was also given a role as a national voice, a right for which CHCs campaigned hard. It was able to put forward the views of patients and the public, including undertaking reviews of policies and services.

The transition

Most of the concerns in Parliament now moved to how the transition would be managed. The transition advisory board (TAB) held its first meeting in February 2002. It was to advise on the implementation of the new arrangements until the establishment of the Commission.[18] Paul Streets, Chief Executive of Diabetes UK, was appointed as Chair. The TAB included representatives from local government, the Commission for Health Improvement, the NHS Confederation, as well as CHCs and the voluntary sector. Of the 17 members, six came from CHCs, two specifically representing staff, though staff issues were outside the remit of the TAB. ACHCEW saw this as attempt to undermine it and divide CHCs, exploiting the increasingly bitter splits within CHCs, in particular between ACHCEW and the Society of CHC Staff. The author was appointed as an external project manager. Department of Health officials did not have the capacity to support the Board and they felt that by appointing an independent person, thought to be acceptable to CHCs and the voluntary sector, the transition might have a greater chance of success.

The TAB's responsibilities were to advise the Department of Health on the transition (see Box 8.4). Its role was not to question the wisdom of policy but advise on how the policy might be implemented. The board was to begin setting initial criteria and standards for the work that the new bodies would undertake. This would provide the Commission with a base from which to

---

Box 8.4   Terms of reference of the transition advisory board

Areas on which the board was to advise included:

- Ensuring a consistent approach to helping CHC lay members and staff to identify opportunities in the new arrangements;
- Ensuring that the new systems built on the best of CHCs;
- Harnessing the skills and experience of CHC members and staff; and
- Advising on the process of setting up and recruiting for the new Commission for Patient and Public Involvement in Health, including developing interim standards in advance of the Commission, and designing its own exit strategy to ensure a smooth handover to the new Commission.

---

start work and it would be able to review and refine standards on a rolling basis.

The TAB started work while the legislation was still going through Parliament. From the start it decided to work in a transparent way with a separate section on the Department of Health's website, where minutes and working group reports were published within days of the meetings and people were able to comment. It also set up a series of consultation events to report on how the new arrangements might work out. This was a different way of working for civil servants. According to one senior civil servant: '*[The TAB] was a genuine attempt to move from the anger of the past year and history into something new and tried to engage with all sides. It nearly drowned civil servants! The minutes of all meetings were posted on the website within 48 hours and were widely read. The Department of Health had never worked in that way before*' (Hogg, 2006b).

The TAB became caught in ACHCEW's battles to amend the legislation. This caused tensions within the TAB where some members felt that ACHCEW was using it to fight a rearguard action that was seen to be increasingly counter-productive. The TAB became marginalised, as if in a parallel universe. While the TAB was considering the functions and staffing establishments for the new Commission and whether the office should be located in or outside London, it emerged that the Department had already identified an office in Birmingham for the Commission and civil servants were choosing the colour for the paintwork. In spite of all this, TAB members were committed and worked hard in four main working groups, largely in agreement. The TAB saw its role as helping the new Commission to be effective. It was aware that if it did not deliver quickly what the Government wanted, the Commission would be vulnerable. The TAB produced an interim report in July 2002 and a final report in December (TAB, 2002a; TAB 2002b).

In July 2002 David Lammy replaced Hazel Blears as minister with responsibility for patient and public involvement. The chair designate for the new Commission, Sharon Grant, was appointed at the end of July 2002. She was a surprise appointment. She had been a Haringey councillor but had no experience in the NHS, user involvement in health or of working at a national level. She had hoped to take over as MP for Tottenham following the death of her husband, Bernie Grant, but David Lammy had been selected instead after a bitter local battle. She was, it seems, placed on the shortlist at the request of the Minister, though she was appointed on her own merits. In reality applications for both chair, commissioners and senior staff positions were limited since there was reluctance to appoint people connected with CHCs. The decision, made by Hazel Blears, to place the headquarters in Birmingham proved critical as it was interpreted by national voluntary organisations and others to mean that the Commission was not taken seriously by the Government. This was not a reflection on Birmingham but on the way power was seen to centre on London. As a result chief executives in the voluntary sector lost interest. They had careers in London and the South East and the Commission no longer looked like a good career move.

The TAB hoped that the Chair Designate would look at it as a shadow commission as she would be working for six months without any commissioners. Immediately it was clear that she had her own vision and wanted a fresh start. The Department of Health also seemed to have lost interest and wanted to leave any decisions to the new Commission as they made clear in the response to the TAB's interim report.[19] The TAB Chair and members discussed privately whether they should close down at that time. However, regional consultation events had been already set up around the country to discuss the recommendations of the TAB. To cancel these would have given the message that the new Commission was not interested in their views and would have set the Commission off to a bad start. It seemed better to carry on. Though the TAB continued until December, the enthusiasm had gone.[20] In spite of the fact that the members of the TAB included some of the most experienced national players in patient and public involvement, none were appointed as Commissioners.

In its interim report the TAB recommended that there should be transition planning in strategic health authority areas. The Department of Health wrote in September 2002 to strategic health authorities to ask them to convene a change action group, involving stakeholders and CHCs, to look at how forums might be configured in their area.[21] The groups' key purpose was to collect local information to inform the Commission's decisions on the establishment of patients' forums, how they might work, including information about how members might be recruited, the location of offices and how staff might be deployed. They were to report to the Commission by 10 January 2003. Many produced reports and worked hard towards this but the reports were apparently not used by CPPIH.

In retrospect the TAB proved an interesting exercise but was ineffective. A civil servant commented that there were too many vested interests on the TAB: '*Ministers did not want what the TAB wanted and the [CPPIH] Chair wanted to go her own way*' (Hogg, 2006f). Another civil servant had a more favourable verdict on the TAB: '[*The Commission] could have run with the agenda set by the TAB and could have had quick wins. For whatever reason the chair took a different view. If other things had gone differently I think that we would have looked back at the TAB as a good system of change management*' (Hogg, 2006b).

The TAB was an attempt to achieve some consensus and carry the voluntary sector and others along with the changes. The appointment of an independent project manager gave the TAB more credibility among the voluntary sector and CHCs and members had more control. However, if ACHCEW had run the TAB, as initially planned, the transition might have been better. It would have kept ACHCEW inside rather than outside the loop. As one member of the ACHCEW management committee observed: '*If ACHCEW had been running the TAB, we would have had to thrash out our differences in private rather than in public. We probably would have got levels of technical agreement quickly and this would have made it harder for ACHCEW to argue substantively*' (Hogg, 2006g).

Instead Ministers and civil servants had become increasingly exasperated with ACHCEW and increasingly unwilling to negotiate. As relations with ACHCEW worsened, the Department of Health was less interested in achieving consensus and transition than in just getting rid of CHCs. This was very frustrating for CHC staff and members, though few thought the new legislation an improvement, many were trying to explore how to make the new arrangements work. The hope was that CPPIH would have influence with the government and be able to get changes to make the system work better and would have the power to ensure more consistency and promote standards among forums – a role that ACHCEW could not take on.

At an ACHCEW special general meeting in July 2003 to wind up the Association, no one from the Government or the Department of Health attended and there was no message of thanks to CHC members who had worked voluntarily for 30 years. CHCs were finally abolished on 30 November 2003. ACHCEW had fought a successful campaign and won many battles but they lost the war. It was a sad ending. It also left anger and a sense of disillusionment at local and national levels that was to persist.

Conclusions

The story of the abolition of CHCs veers between tragedy and farce. No one predicted that such a minor part of health policy would cause so much political damage. The case for the reform of CHCs was uncontested, but the case for abolition was not. Was it a conspiracy or a cock-up? Undoubtedly, it started as a conspiracy to make sure that the news of the abolition of CHCs was not leaked before the announcement. But what followed was a cock-up based on misunderstandings, obstinacy and personality clashes, rather than issues of principle. The end result was unworkable legislation, a complex and fragmented system and failure to learn from 30 years' experience of user involvement. Many of those who supported the abolition from the start recognise that, in retrospect, reform would have been better.

This story also gives an interesting insight into policy-making. It illustrates the basic problems with democracy highlighted in the Power Inquiry (2006). Decisions that fundamentally affected many people were made in secrecy without consultation. It showed how powerful ministers had become compared to

MPs and how far the traditional role of civil servants had been undermined by political advisers. The resulting lack of openness and transparency led to poor decision-making.

Did the Government want to divide and fragment the voice of patients and the public in order to reduce opposition to their national policies, as some commentators have suggested? (Milewa et al., 2003). Was it an attempt to divert community and patient activism into local consumerist issues of quality and access rather than broader public engagement? Whatever the intention, without CHCs the introduction of radical changes in healthcare was made easier for the Government. ACHCEW with its well informed briefing papers and national networks might have activated more widespread opposition amongst the voluntary sector against the reforms.

But there were losses for local communities. CHCs had increasingly become the organisational memory for local health services. Throughout the reorganisations of the NHS over 25 years, CHCs remained a constant local focal point. CHCs were able to follow up issues which were otherwise forgotten. With the abolition of CHCs, this organisational memory was lost. In a research study commissioned by the Department of Health on public involvement, a member of the public interviewed summarised this: '*There have been quite a number of consultations, forums, get-togethers and reports and it's put on file... Then, a few years later on you are asked exactly the same questions again and part of the reason is because the statutory bodies are always restructuring and reports get lost and have to start all over again*' (Farrell, 2004: 32).

CHCs clearly needed reform but the costs of abolition were high. Peter Walsh summed this up: '*What we have lost with CHCs is the local watchdog, something tangible which was really important for communities. It was really important for communities to feel they had their own CHC. Now we have a vague process, not a body or institution that you can identify with. Even the very few weak or ineffective CHCs did some good and did no harm. Where they worked well, they were fantastic*' (Hogg, 2006h).

The Second Coming – The Commission and Patients' Forums

'*When governments replace one grassroots organisation with what they say is another, they shouldn't be surprised if the people become suspicious. So, this second coming for "patient power" has not been greeted with unalloyed enthusiasm.*' Geoff Watts, *British Medical Journal*, 326, 8 March 2003.

Overview

This chapter looks at the work of Commission for Patient and Public Involvement in Health (CPPIH) and the reasons for its short life.
- CPPIH started work in difficult circumstances.
- Its abolition was announced within 18 months and the abolition of patients' forums two years later.
- Among the reasons for failure was the reluctance to learn from the experiences of CHCs and the lack of political will at national level to make the new arrangements work.

This chapter is based on interviews with key participants in these events as part of a research study.

Introduction

By autumn 2002 the legislation was passed in England, the Chair of CPPIH had been appointed and the process of appointing the chief executive and commissioners was beginning. In strategic health authorities change action groups were drawing up information on each area to help the Commission plan. During the passage of the legislation ACHCEW had achieved three promises from the Government: that the new PCT forums would be one-stop shops, that CHCs would not be abolished until the new systems were properly functioning, and an implied promise that there would be some transition for staff and members. ACHCEW had accepted that they were going and wanted a role in the transition. Many CHCs were setting up pilot forums;

Box 9.1   The rise and fall of the Commission for Patient and Public Involvement in Health

May 2002 – NHS and Healthcare Professions Act passed.

July 2002 – Chair Designate appointed.

January 2003 – CPPIH formally starts work.

March 2003 – First Board meeting held in public.

April 2003 – CPPIH announces forum support to be contracted to external agencies

September 2003 – Recruitment of members starts.

30 November – CHCs and ACHCEW abolished.

December 2003 – Patients' forums established.

July 2004 – Arms Length Review recommends the abolition of CPPIH.

May 2006 – Report of expert panel published.

July 2006 – Abolition of Patients' forums announced.

July 2006 – Department of Health publishes 'A Stronger Voice'.

February 2007 – House of Commons Health Committee report on patient and public involvement published.

October 2007 – Local Government of Public Involvement Act passed.

31 March 2008 – CPPIH and patients' forums abolished.

1 April 2008 – Local involvement networks set up.

---

some funded by the Department of Health, and were recruiting and training new people who had not previously been involved in CHCs.[1,2]

However, the Commission had its own vision and approached its task in a way that ministers and civil servants had not anticipated. A summary of events is outlined in Box 9.1. Changes in other UK countries are described in Chapter 10.

Battles commence

The Commission, even before it was set up, had been dealt a bad hand. The new system of patient and public involvement was criticised for its complexity and incoherence (Baggott, 2005). The House of Commons Health Select Committee warned in 2003 that the '*confusion at the launch of a system may erode the public's confidence in it, meaning that it has failed before it has started*' (2003: 9). The circumstances of its creation meant that there was scepticism amongst the voluntary sector at local and national levels. The Government too seemed to have lost interest. 'Choice' now had more priority in national policy than 'voice'. In December 2002 it was announced that the planned foundation hospitals were to have no patients' forums and that in time all trusts would become foundation trusts. Plans were in place to make forums redundant before they were set up.

A difficult task was made almost impossible for the Commission by the time-scale imposed by the Government. In response to backbench pressure ministers had promised that CHCs would not be abolished until arrangements to take over their functions were in place. On 4 June 2003 David Lammy, the Minister, announced that CHCs' life would be extended to 30 November 2003 and that forums would be established by then. This was a blow for the Commission which had assumed that it had until April 2004 to set up the new arrangements, but now forums were to be in place four months earlier. The Commission was given no time to set itself up or understand the tasks it had to do.

Then new battles started. The first battle was with the Department of Health over the budget allocated to the Commission, the next with ACHCEW and CHC staff over the decision to contract out the staffing of forums to the voluntary sector. These were followed by internal battles about the vision and the management of the organisation.

The budget

The first battle was over the budget. The Transition Advisory Board (TAB) had been informed that the overall budget would be in the region of £29 million, but the Commission wanted an annual budget of £64 million.[3] This would have enabled a similar level of resources for each forum as CHCs had had. In comparison to the budget for CHCs, the Commission had an additional £11 million but it felt this was not enough to run forums as well as its other responsibilities. The Chair and Chief Executive were successful in arguing for more money and the budget and strategy was finally agreed in April 2003 at £34.5 million. Although achieving a £5 million increase in the budget was significant, many members of the Board believed that too many compromises would have to be made. But the negotiation process had already delayed the start of the work and antagonised ministers and civil servants. This affected the reputation of the Commission, as it launched itself into the public arena.

The Commission had made enemies before it had made any friends. It was not a good start.

Staff support for forums

In November 2002 the new Chief Executive, Laura McMurtrie, joined the Commission from the NHS. By then the decision to start from scratch had been made. This meant that it would not be possible to develop transition arrangements for CHC staff. The Chief Executive was disappointed that there would be no opportunity to try to merge the two systems, believing that CHC experience and the goodwill towards them would be lost, and this would damage CPPIH as it sought to establish an identity (Hogg, 2007a). However, others in the Commission and the Department of Health felt that patients' forums were expected to operate fundamentally differently from CHCs and that support from CHCs would limit the Commission's opportunity to establish new ways of working.

The Chief Executive then suggested that forums be based around local authority areas which provided social services, and had overview and scrutiny committees. However, lawyers advised that ministers had intended that 572 forums be set up and that this would not reflect the will of Parliament. The Department of Health was insistent that the number of forums should follow the legislation – a separate forum for every NHS trust and PCT.

If it was not possible to build the new system on CHCs, the Chief Executive felt that the next best was to take advantage of the existing voluntary sector infrastructure and contract voluntary organisations to provide staff support for 150 local networks of forums, matching local government areas. This would enable the Commission to establish itself quickly, gain the benefit of existing knowledge and networks, and avoid developing its own bureaucracy (Hogg, 2007a). The decision to contract out staff support for forums to local network providers was taken by the Chair on the advice of the Chief Executive and put to the first full meeting of the commissioners. It was to have far reaching implications.

The backlash

The predicted backlash happened when CPPIH announced that it would not directly employ staff, but advertise for voluntary and non-profit organisations to bid for contracts to support patients' forums. CHC staff had assumed that they would be given first choice of posts in the new bodies or, at least, fair access. However, it now emerged that this was not the intention. If forums were considered in any way as a continuation of CHCs, CHC staff would have had rights under the Transfer of Undertakings (Protection of Employment) Regulations 1981 (TUPE). This was not what the Commission or Department of Health apparently wanted. The Commission did not enter into discussions with ACHCEW in case by implication any employment rights were given to staff. The Chief Executive reported to the Board that it was difficult to have a dialogue with CHCs during the transition period as the Commission did not have the capacity to do this.[4] A CHC chief officer on the ACHCEW management committee summed up the mood in the spring of 2003: '*There was a feeling of betrayal and worthlessness. We had been doing things we were committed to and felt were really worthwhile and we were being cast aside with no obvious alternative to replace us. If CHCs were to have been replaced with something better, it would have been easier*' (Hogg, 2006i).

ACHCEW then turned against the Commission. A member of the ACHCEW management committee reported: '*Once it was clear that [the Department of Health] had broken the terms of the agreement, we were entitled to revert to an oppositional role and therefore gave them a hard time*' (Hogg, 2006g). Malcolm Alexander, Chief Officer of Southwark CHC, was appointed as acting director. ACHCEW was back campaigning – what it did best. Legal advice sought by ACHCEW advised that the contracting arrangement proposed might be unlawful, while legal advice to the Department of Health and CPPIH advised otherwise. The Commission felt under attack. In July 2003 a meeting of the All-Party Parliamentary Group on CHCs, for which ACHCEW provided the secretariat, excluded ACHCEW at the request of CPPIH.[5]

ACHCEW continued to embarrass the government. In March 2003 David Lammy told the House of Commons Select Committee that 96 per-cent of trusts had patient advice and liaison services, though the information was not collected centrally. ACHCEW carried out a survey which cast doubt on this claim (ACHCEW, 2003). When the Health Select Committee looked at patient and public involvement in May 2003, David Lammy, the Minister, was heavily criticised in their report for his *'failure to grasp the subtle but extremely important distinctions between the organisations his government is currently setting up'* (House of Commons Select Committee, 2003, Para 26). Before the report was published he moved to the Department of Constitutional Affairs and was replaced by Rosie Winterton as the Minister responsible for patient and public involvement.

Debates in the House of Lords

It was not only ACHCEW that was angry about the proposed local network providers. It was not what Parliament or the Department of Health had intended. Questions were regularly asked in Parliament, mainly on the transition for CHCs. Conservative MP Stephen O'Brien complained that the Commission would not engage with CHCs. He complained that at a stakeholders' meeting involving the Department of Health, ACHCEW, CHCs and trade unions, CPPIH chair did not turn up. Instead, the Commission sent along someone who had been in her job for only eight days. *'What sort of commitment'*, he asked, *'does that reveal on the part of a Government-created commission to deliver on the Government's promise to learn from the knowledge of CHCs' experienced staff?'*[6]

Tabling Regulations is generally a formality, but a motion to remit can force a debate. There were debates in the House of Lords in February and October 2003. The main concerns were that promises made by Ministers in order to get the legislation passed had not been observed by the Commission. The new forums were not to be one-stop shops and there was to be no smooth transition from the old to the new arrangements. Lord Clement Jones, for the Liberal Democrats, suggested that the Department of Health was deliberately constructing a system designed to exclude CHC staff and there was a deliberate desire to manipulate them out of the system. Earl Howe, the Conservative health spokesman, expressed dismay that the assurances received from Ministers for a seamless transition from the old arrangements to the new had counted for nothing. *'The abandonment of ministerial undertakings, on the strength of which amendments to last year's legislation were withdrawn, is an extremely serious matter...... Ministers do take decisions, but they should also abide by the assurances that they have previously given.'*[7] Earl Howe concluded that *'It is a very grave list of charges and one is tempted to conclude that the whole system has been set up to fail'*.[8]

The contracting process

The contracting process for local network providers soon ran into practical difficulties. The chief executive obtained legal advice that the commissioners should be excluded from the contracting process because of the potential conflict of interest as they had close links with the voluntary sector. As a result commissioners were not involved in drawing up service specifications or awarding contracts. There was a difference of opinion between board members and the executive team on this, which continued into the following year. To some commissioners it felt like they had responsibility without authority. The commissioners reluctantly accepted their exclusion, though when the renewal of contracts came up in 2006, there was no objection to their involvement. The exclusion of the commissioners, with their experience and understanding of the voluntary sector and the NHS, was unfortunate. Their advice might have been useful since the contract team was made up of temporary staff from a consulting firm and most had no experience of the voluntary sector, the NHS or patient and public involvement. Some contracts were awarded to local networks where boundaries were not co-terminous and did not reflect local communities or health economies. This was to make co-operation between PPI forums harder to achieve.

Controversy increased when the contracts were announced. Many of the organisations appointed had little experience of patient advocacy or the NHS. Some, such as Age Concern or SCOPE, had expertise limited to specific areas of health policy. Others, such as Scout Enterprises, had no links with health. Many providers were also not local. Scout Enterprises administered 20 forums in Berkshire, Hampshire, Bristol and Cornwall and was based in Bristol. SCOPE was based in Birmingham and provided administration for forums in South London. Local networks providers were then renamed forum support organisations (FSOs). Inevitably in some areas there were no bidders and the Commission had to ask some contractors to take on forums and areas that they had not tendered for. The choice of contractor caused division and resentment in some areas where an external organisation with no particular interest in health or link with that community was taking over from the local CHC, most of which were embedded in the local voluntary sector. In some areas local councils of voluntary service had tendered to be the support organisations but were not successful and an outside agency had been brought in. There was a perception in the voluntary sector that some organisations were using contracts to finance other activities (Hogg, 2004). There were also concerns about the viability and suitability of some of the network providers. One of them, the College of Health went into voluntary liquidation within weeks of the start of the contract. There were particular concerns with the Haringey-based Community Investors Development Agency (CIDA) which provided support to 15 forums in North London. The Chief Executive of Haringey Council wrote to the Commission saying that the Council would not be confident of being able to work constructively with CIDA. CIDA threatened the Chief Executive with legal action unless he apologised and paid his staff compensation.[9] When the contracts came up for renewal nine of the 68 organisations covering 126 forums did not continue.[10]

The vision

The Commission was to have a role wider than setting up and managing patients' forums – now renamed patient and public involvement (PPI) forums and ICAS. It was to promote patient and public involvement in the NHS and be a national voice, undertaking reviews of policies and services. However, pressure to set up forums quickly meant the Commission was expected to perform its functions before it had the chance to reflect on the nature of its role or establish itself. Perhaps, as a result, from the start there seemed to be no shared vision for the Commission, but several visions.

The Department of Health wanted the Commission and forums to engage with the NHS, bringing user involvement into clinical governance. It wanted the Commission to advise the NHS on how they could involve patients and public better and to promote good practice. The Commission, on the other hand, interpreted the legislation to be to be about public health, long-term culture change and democratisation.[11] The Commission felt that the Department of Health was compromising its ability to respond to the wider policy challenges of public engagement by concentrating too much of its resources on inspection and compliance. The need to deliver the quick short-term gains that politicians wanted rather than focus on longer-term objectives was a tension for the emerging visions and priorities of CPPIH.

'*Our Health*' was the Chair's vision. It was an attempt to tie forums into the wider citizenship agenda by enabling people, who did not want to be forum members, to get involved on their own terms. Regional managers were encouraged to recruit people who were interested in health issues and would be prepared to comment by phone, post or online. However, it was not possible for CPPIH to take '*Our Health*' forward because of more urgent demands on resources and it was dropped in March 2004.

The Chief Executive looked to technological solutions. Since the new system was potentially fragmented, she thought the answer was to link the 572 forums and their local network providers together with a computer network.[12] The vision for the Knowledge Management System (KMS) was a website where people could find, discuss and share information on health issues and the activities of forums. The network could also bring a whole range of information to the public to see how they could contribute and find health information, providing the information base for future citizen engagement, as envisaged by the Wanless Report. Some commissioners were sceptical about the benefits of such a major financial investment and it took up a large proportion of the first year's budget, with dedicated staff in each regional office employed to input data. By 2006 it cost £500,000 a year to run. However, it had not been developed with its users and never reached its potential.

The commissioners were people with expertise in user involvement and had their own vision. One commissioner expressed it thus: '*We, the commissioners, wanted a movement for social change, building something that was sustainable and rooted in communities. But this was seen as woolly thinking by the management team. The Department of Health and the Chair wanted a top-down organisation. Commissioners did not necessarily want forums but networks and build these up from a collective base, but it was soon totally out of control*' (Hogg, 2006j).

Being forced to work under so much pressure, it was not surprising that relationships broke down and internally the organisation soon became fragmented. The relationship between the Chair and Chief Executive deteriorated, causing internal difficulties for those working in the organisation who felt that they did not know who was ultimately in charge.

The first CPPIH Board meeting was held in public in March 2003. In the first year, the meetings attracted up to 80 people, mainly from CHCs. With so much, often hostile, scrutiny, the commissioners were expected to show a united front. To the outside world the commissioners seemed quiet and unforthcoming with no sense of their own importance. The public meetings were '*staged and showcased*', according to one commissioner (Hogg, 2006j). Admission tickets had to be obtained in advance.

There were tensions and conflict between the commissioners and the management team from early on. Most of the staff had no background in the voluntary sector or user involvement, while the commissioners did not have experience of running large public bodies and none were from the major voluntary organisations or had a national profile. A commissioner identified a clash of cultures and values between the public and voluntary sectors that undermined the organisation. Public sector experience was more valued than expertise in patient and public involvement or voluntary sector experience. There was a policy to match the terms of service for any person recruited from the public sector to get the 'best' people. This was not offered to people from the voluntary sector. As a commissioner observed: '*The management team was completely process-driven and focused on delivering targets. Risk, finance, and facilities dominated the board meetings. There was no room for proper debate about what we were trying to achieve and how we could get there. The management team lacked any understanding about what they were doing... Several occasions we were told that legal advice meant we could not do something we wanted to do. It was completely the wrong approach, but to them it was how you dealt with a perceived problem and was quite logical*' (Hogg, 2006k).

Commissioners had already been excluded from the strategic decisions, and now they found their expertise in user involvement was not called upon. One commissioner summed it up: '*At the start I was hugely enthusiastic and increasingly feeling the need to work from within as well as from outside. This was finally the possibility to get formal recognition for user involvement and community development as part of the NHS... Within six months we felt it was getting away from us, always troubleshooting and never getting hold of what we were trying to achieve*' (Hogg, 2006j).

The Commission, which had a difficult task in the best of times, was under attack before it had really got started. As the criticisms mounted, the

Commission became increasingly introverted. As one commissioner said: *'There was a siege mentality within the Commission. The ultimate enemy was always the Department of Health'* (Hogg, 2006j).

Recruiting members

The Chair on the advice of the Chief Executive had decided to recommend to the Board setting up nine regional offices to *'directly support forums by providing advice and guidance, supporting the sharing of information, learning and development, communications, accessibility, governance and FSO contract compliance'*.[13] Each regional office was given an establishment of 17 staff, though the number of forums they were responsible for varied from 30 in the North East to 93 in the South East. Regional offices with staff and premises were set up in a short time. The Commission was proud of this achievement. A commissioner pointed out that this infrastructure, including patch technology for transferring telephone callers to offices across the whole of the country, was to become the envy of other arms length bodies – most of which had been established for longer than CPPIH.

Having set up the regional offices and contracted local network providers, the Commission set out to recruit members and set standards for their work and activities. The Commission was faced with a great challenge to recruit 7000–12,000 members, 12–20 for each forum. Recognising the monumental task of recruiting forum members and the importance of continuity and 'organisational memory', the TAB had emphasised the importance of local connections in recruitment and suggested that CHCs should get involved in helping to recruit interested people during their last days. By the middle of 2003 there were still about 4000 CHC members (about 1000 vacancies out of 5000 places). ACHCEW estimated that about 1500 CHC members, perhaps with training for the new role, would be interested in becoming forum members and the TAB suggested they could provide a core for the new forums. It also suggested that PCT Forums should be set up first and they could then assist in setting up forums in NHS trusts. In many areas CHCs working with trusts had set up 'shadow' forums or panels, anticipating the changes and in the expectation that they would then transfer to the new arrangements when established. A staged approach would be easier for CPPIH to oversee and enable it to learn from experience (TAB, 2002b).

However, the Commission did not want to transfer members from CHCs or work with the remaining CHCs to recruit members and set up forums. The Commission chose a national campaign. The slogan was *You Don't Need to Wear a Chicken Suit and Run a Marathon to Be Interested in Health*. Regional offices were issued with a chicken suit which they were encouraged to use to recruit members off the street. It was the first time since 1974 that a nationally co-ordinated advertising campaign (with adverts appearing on buses and the underground) had been used to seek patient and public involvement. However, it did not go down well with many CPPIH staff or the NHS. At a national conference an eminent policy analyst held the state of patient and public involvement up to ridicule. We had the dog (a reference to ACHCEW's demonstrations in dog costumes outside Parliament) and now we have the chicken, he said.

Recruitment of members started in September 2003. Though the contracts of FSOs had commenced on 1 September, they were not required to assist in the recruitment of members. Teams from a commercial consulting firm moved into the regional offices to organise the recruitment. Most did not have a background in the voluntary sector or an understanding of volunteers. One regional manager was concerned about the process, reporting that they rejected some applicants because their first language was not English or they were seen to have poor literacy. Some regional office staff took stalls in local events and got people to fill in forms, interviewed and signed them up there and then. By mid-November it was agreed that regional staff could do telephone interviews. This was quicker but it meant that the new forum members had little briefing and did not know what they were committing themselves to do before they turned up at the first formal meeting. In the end the regional staff were cold calling potential recruits in the evening and weekends and signing up their friends and relations in order to meet the deadline. At the start it had been hoped to exclude those with prior involvement but by November anyone who applied was appointed (Hogg, 2006l; 2006m).

Individuals were recruited, rather than representatives of voluntary organisations, though this was specified in legislation. A regional manager reported: '*The Commission did not encourage the appointment of members with links in the community or the recruitment of people from voluntary organisations. They did not understand that there might be different arrangements for the recruitment of individuals from voluntary organisations and those recruited as individuals and there was no guidance on their role as members of networks...Members of the executive team were anti-CHC and this attitude permeated throughout the whole organisation. They were obstinate in their refusal to learn from CHCs*' (Hogg, 2006l). Little thought was given to how members would be 'representative' or relate to their constituencies, undermining any claims to legitimacy.

Against the odds the Commission had met the deadline and recruited over 4000 members by 30 November 2003.[14] Each forum had the legal minimum number of seven members. Those involved in the Government at the time recognise in retrospect that by putting so much pressure to set up forums by 1 December 2003 was unrealistic. A civil servant noted: '*If the Commission had had six months longer it might have been very different and they could have developed criteria and a clearer idea of the role for members*' (Hogg, 2006f). The pressure meant that priority was given to getting names rather than the making sure the people recruited were suitable and understood their role.

Forums, support organisations and the Commission

Forums were slow to get started. The number of forums caused confusion. Some NHS trust forums covered services provided to several different PCTs.

Most forums only had a handful of members. They had no local office and limited staff support. A survey in the Health Service Journal in April 2004 found that many forums were already struggling to survive due to lack of resources and poor administrative support.[15] As the emphasis was on recruiting people new to volunteering, user advocacy and the NHS, forum members required more rather than less staff support than CHC members, most of whom were already associated with other organisations in the community. A regional manager described it thus: '*For new members it was very confusing; they got their appointment letter that had very little briefing about what being a member involved and then there was no follow up until they received a letter from the forum support organisation inviting them to the first meeting, which would be on a completely different headed paper. Often the initial meetings were difficult with staff who knew nothing about PPI, the NHS or the local area and had no relationship with the organisation to which they had been appointed [CPPIH]. We suggested to people who were interested in becoming members that they should attend the forum meeting, but those that did found them a shambles and did not join*' (Hogg, 2006l).

The complex three tier structure meant there was great scope for misunderstandings and disputes. Soon the Commission came under attack from forums and blamed for the problems. Though forum members were public appointments, their names could not be divulged even to other members because they had not given their consent under the Data Protection Act. This was not a good start either in public accountability or in helping forum members to get to know each other and work together. The Commission communicated with forums through FSOs but this was variable so that communication with forums was unpredictable. Therefore the Commission related to individual forum members rather than to forums as corporate bodies. Later they gained information on policy issues from members through '60 second' online polls and gained feedback on the performance of FSOs through surveys of individual members rather than asking the forum as a whole.[16]

The national centre in Birmingham was reluctant to delegate powers to the regional offices. If the regional office had a query from the FSO about buying an aid for someone with a disability, there was no policy and this was referred to the head office. A regional manager reported: '*The way decisions were taken was hierarchical and not consultative. There was no one in the senior management team who had experience or understanding of the voluntary sector or PPI. At senior management team meetings, the executives at headquarters would present their proposals, and the regional officers would complain that they were not consulted. There was no understanding about the ways to work with volunteers. You cannot give them directions without involving or consulting them*' (Hogg, 2006l).

Relationships between the national centre and some forums became acrimonious and continued to be so.[17,18] One contentious area was always money. Because FSOs did not have a budget to pay for travel, there were difficulties in the early days for members claiming travel expenses. There was further anger when members found that they were being offered a lower mileage rate than senior managers. Forum budgets were also a problem. The legislation required forums to take responsibility for their budgets and sign an annual financial report. However, the Commission did not allocate budgets to individual forums and they were not allowed to know how much the FSO contract was for their forum. As a result to comply with legislation, forums were required to sign a nil return each year.

In practice regional offices spent a lot of time dealing with problems of individual members and there were few ways of ensuring that other members did not act in a discriminatory or racist manner. A regional manager observed: *'Because of the speed of the recruitment, with just a short interview there was no opportunity to assess the skills or aptitude of the members who were first appointed. Some had no idea how to work in a group or to be accountable. We had to take several through the standards committee, as their behaviour was inappropriate, for example racist, sexist or acting alone or contacting the media without the agreement of the forum'* (Hogg, 2006l). Alternative websites were set up by forum members and one was closed down following the threat of legal action by the Commission for defamation.[19] Some members resigned because they felt that the regional office did not support them in disputes with their FSO and a database of 'victims' was set up – forum members who felt that they had been harassed or victimised by CPPIH or their FSO.[20]

The nature of the relationship between staff and members was very different from CHCs. CHC members chose and managed their own staff, who were employed by the NHS. Forums had no choice in either the FSO or the staff provided for them. Accountability of the FSO was to the Commission and not to the forum. In trying to get away from the formality of CHCs, forums were not required to have a chair though most did. With no leadership, forums ran into difficulties and disputes between members who had little support and guidance and no staff to mediate or defuse situations. The chair of the CHC was formally elected annually and had more status and so was in a position to mediate in disputes among members or between members and staff.

In 2004 many of the fresh recruits lapsed and many resigned because of the lack of support they received. Recruitment and retention remained problematic, with a reported 11 percent of PPI forum members resigning within the first six months of their appointment.[21] CHCs in 1975 faced the same problem when members realised they were expected to do more than attend a few meetings. CHC members could be removed by their appointing body if they were inactive for four months. There was no provision for getting rid of inactive forum members; they could only be removed on grounds of misconduct. By the end of 2004 80 forums had fallen below the statutory minimum of seven members, which was far below the expected number of 12–20 per forum.[22]

Performance management

The Commission had been expected to set standards and review the performance of forums, but there was a feeling within the Commission that this was not appropriate and it should not tell forums how to run themselves.[23] A regional manager observed *'there were frequent debates within the Commission about whether they should performance manage forums at all since they were independent'* (Hogg, 2006m). Relationships with forums had got off to a bad start and it was felt that trying to impose performance management at this stage would exacerbate the situation.

Regional offices were responsible for contract and performance management of FSOs and forums. Performance management for FSOs was brought in after the contracts had been issued and performance managers were not recruited until February 2004. Though the contracts with FSOs were confidential, it soon emerged that some FSOs had been given more money than others to provide the same services.[24] This apparent unfairness led to feelings of resentment among FSOs. From the start the role of FSOs had not been clear: who was the servant and who was the master? Was their role just to arrange meetings and type up minutes of meetings or should it be more than this? It was not clear if they could advise members on strategy, help recruit new members or arrange their own training for members.[25] Box 9.2 illustrates these problems.

Verdicts on patients' forums

It is unfair to judge forums since they were not given time to develop and get to grips with their role. They had none of the advantages that CHCs had in 1974. CHC abolition had little support in local communities, and so forums did not inherit any goodwill or meet with local enthusiasm. They had fewer members, less staff support and no separate budget. There were the same structural flaws in forums as in CHCs: the lack of accountability, inconsistencies in their approaches and questions about the legitimacy of members.

However, in spite of all the difficulties many dedicated volunteers worked hard to try and make the system work. The most common areas investigated were infection control, GP services, transport and parking, mental health, community involvement, out-of-hours services, health information, older people services and disability services.[26] There were successes particularly in mental health trusts and in ambulance services, where scrutiny had not been so well developed by CHCs.

For NHS managers, if CHCs had been a side show, forums did not even get to the fair. A survey found that most PCT staff met at least quarterly with forums, but they considered them to be the least likely to be influential in commissioning decisions, less influential than voluntary or patients' groups (Chisholm et al., 2007). In a survey by the *Health Service Journal* only 16 percent of managers responding were confident that forums were up to the job, the rest were unsure or worried. The NHS Confederation took the view that forums were still not sufficiently developed as organisations in all cases to give sophisticated corroborative evidence on the process.[27] When PPI forum members were invited to national events, managers were not impressed. One manager commented: *'Each had a different interpretation of*

Box 9.2   Problems between forums and the Commission

In a London Borough there were particular difficulties between members and the forum support organisation. The forums complained that their forum support organ-isation 'would not accept direction from us. They thought their role was to monitor and check on us.'[28] They also complained about the level of support they were given by their FSO and that they got less than one day's work per week for the £34,000 p.a. that the organisation received. The Chair of the Overview and Scrutiny Committee (OSC) also complained to CIPPIH about the FSO. 'We asked [the FSO] to circulate an invitation to a meeting with the OSC to members of the forums. They said they had no capacity to do this. We then asked for the names of members but they would not give us the names as they said these were not in the public domain. We then offered them the stamped envelopes that they could address and they refused to do this, as it was an intrusion into the privacy of members!' (Hogg, 2006p).

At a meeting convened by CPPIH to discuss the complaint, the FSO informed three forum chairs that they were participating in the meeting without prejudice to legal action. Members saw this as an implied threat of legal action against them personally. CPPIH interpreted the situation differently, seeing it as 'a reasonable statement to make and did not imply or suggest legal action'.[29] However, CPPIH was seen to be siding with the FSO against their own volunteers and several forum members resigned. The chair of the PCT forum observed: 'It comes back to the lack of support from [the FSO] and the whole working relationship. There is a top-heavy bureaucracy by CPPIH which is more inter-ested in control than support' (Hogg, 2006q). The PCT forum unanimously called for an independent investigation into the FSO's work in Camden. An investigation was undertaken by CPPIH and the FSO's contract was not renewed in that Borough.

One particular forum member who caused angst for the national centre was Malcolm Alexander, the last director of ACHCEW and now the Chair of the London Ambulance Service Patients Forum. On an independent website for forum members he said that the Commission had 'a hopeless inexperienced leadership'. He publicly crit-icised the Chair and Chief Executive in a letter to Private Eye by referring to a letter from the Chair defending their record as 'disingenuous'.[30] Malcolm Alexander then received a letter from lawyers Hill Dickinson who threatened to immediately com-mence a high court action for defamation against him in person unless he made a public apology. Instead he passed it on to Private Eye who repeated the defamatory comments since, as they said, they had more resources and more robust lawyers.[31] The criticism seemed to be within the range of fair comment about public figures and taking legal action to suppress such comments might be considered an inappropriate use of public funds. It was also naïve. Such actions are more likely to inflame than intimidate community activists.

---

the world, they had small numbers of members and some had a very limited knowledge of the health service. I went away saddened from the meeting, thinking that we had lost a lot when we lost the organisational memory of CHCs. And we had just gone back to scratch' (Hogg, 2007b).

The Healthcare Commission used patients' forums to help them assess whether trusts were meeting their core standards. In this they found that forums did not always perform well, as a manager there observed: '*Very early on it was clear that – although some forums did a sterling job – others were falling into the trap that CHCs fell into: instead of enabling people to become involved, they acted as a barrier and were encouraged to think they were "it". ......They did not necessarily have the skills to involve other people and some developed a victim mentality, thinking of themselves (not unreasonably) as under appreciated, sometimes neglected outsiders*' (Hogg, 2006n).

The impact of PPI forums generally was limited. They were largely invisible in their communities. Members had no formal links to the local authority or the voluntary sector, and so were more peripheral to the politics of the local health economy. They were not appointed or elected by local bodies and did not have their own office with staff. For a member of the public to contact their local PPI forum was not straightforward. They had to find out who the FSO was and contact them, and they might not be based in the locality. The names and addresses of PPI forum members were not publicly available. Meetings did not have to be held in public and papers were not available to the public. In contrast CHC members' names and addresses were publicly available and they were required to advertise and hold meetings in public and make all their papers and working documents available to the public.

Building a national movement

The hope for the Commission was that it would provide leadership for the user movement, bringing together at national level the voluntary sector and forums and ensure that those involved felt part of a wider movement where they were valued and had something to contribute. However, there is a contradiction for a top-down organisation appointed by government becoming a voice for users. Non-departmental public bodies, like the Commission, are, by definition, top-down organisations, with commissioners appointed who meet the criteria of the great and good. The Department of Health had proposed that the commissioners should mainly be people working at local level with relevant expertise (DH, 2001b). The TAB suggested that: '*There is an exciting opportunity to develop new forms of governance that are more inclusive and ensure that people involved at local level feel that they have a stake at national level*' (TAB, 2002b). The TAB discussed this with the NHS Appointments Commission who agreed that there could be different ways of appointing commissioners. While the first commissioners would be appointed by the NHS Appointments Commission for practical reasons, there could be elections at a later stage.

The TAB proposed that there should be regional assemblies for forums based on the nine government regions that would advise on regional and cross-boundary issues and specialist services and feed in experiences from forums and ICAS to national policy. The Commission's regional offices did not necessarily see their role to encourage forums to get together. London forums set up a network with the support of the regional office, but most regions did not. The commissioners were, for a period, allocated a regional responsibility. A commissioner said: *'Though this looked good on paper, it was never clear what the role of the regional commissioner was. For several of the commissioners the role became to act as an advocate for the staff in the regional centre who wanted to get their issues at the top of the agenda'* (Hogg, 2006k).

The annual conference was an important event in the calendar for CHCs. It provided support, enabled networking for staff and members, allowed CHCs to showcase their work and gave them a sense of being part of a national movement. In July 2005 a national convention for PPI forums was held in Birmingham. This was largely seen as a success, but was not repeated. The Department of Health was not enthusiastic and did not agree this as part of the workplan for the following year.

Some forum members wanted to set up a national association that could speak for them. With the abolition of the Commission, a national network was urgently needed to enable members to have a say in the arrangements that were to be made for them following the abolition of CPPIH. In a workshop at the national convention, it was agreed by those present that they would like a national association and the Commission agreed to convene the working group. In September 2005 the Commission asked members for their views and for nominations for a steering group to look at how an association might be set up. The Commission provided administrative support to the steering group and agreed to arrange elections for the management committee in April 2006. However, nothing further happened and the abolition of forums was announced in June 2006. The elections eventually took place in March 2007 once legislation was already going through Parliament and too late to have an impact. In May Malcolm Alexander, the last director of ACHCEW, was elected chair of the new national association, perhaps confirming CPPIH's misgivings.

The arms length review and the end

The abolition of CPPIH was announced in July 2004, as part of the review of arms length bodies (DH, 2004b). However well the Commission had performed, it would have been vulnerable as its functions were dispensable. But disillusionment had soon set in with the new arrangements. Forums and CPPIH were not seen as a success and had little visibility (Lewis, 2005a). The Commission had been overwhelmed by the task of setting up forums and this meant that it focussed on internal matters. It had not been given time to settle into its role or make alliances at national or grass roots level. National bodies complained that the Commission did not answer letters and was not prepared to work with them. This had led to the marginalisation of the Commission. The NHS Confederation, having failed to get a meeting with the Commission, turned away from the Commission and forums to focus on other forms of patient and public involvement: foundation trusts, health information and direct working with the public. The All-Party Parliamentary Group on Patient and Public Involvement had 20 members in 2006, compared to the All-Party Group on CHCs that it replaced which had 240 members in 1999. As a result when their abolition was announced, the Commission had made few friends and few voices were raised to defend it.

The review left the Department of Health with a difficulty. Forums were to remain with members appointed by the Appointments Commission. Other functions, such as setting standards and monitoring forums and promoting patient and public involvement within the NHS, would, it was hoped, be passed on to the Healthcare Commission. However, neither the Appointments Commission nor the Healthcare Commission were willing to take on these tasks. To assist in developing detailed proposals, the Department of Health and CPPIH commissioned the author to carry out a survey of the views of national voluntary organisations. Almost 30 people in national organisations involved in patient and public involvement were interviewed. This survey found that there was anger that the Department of Health had reneged on its commitments made during the abolition of CHCs, but little support for the Commission or forums. The Commission was seen as inward-looking and bureaucratic.[32] There was also criticism that the provision of staff through external agencies had added an unnecessary tier between staff and forums. Many felt that the CHC model, where staff were employed by the NHS but accountable to the members, had worked well and not jeopardised the CHC's independence.

Rather than carry out a formal consultation based on written proposals, the Department of Health commissioned Opinion Leader Research to undertake a consultation exercise, using 14 deliberative workshops with forum members, FSOs and CPPIH staff and an online survey (OLR, 2005). The method of consultation was egalitarian but not deliberative. It gave equal weight to the views of a member of the public unfamiliar with the issue and a national voluntary organisation representing many members. Over 4000 online questionnaires were returned. Over two-thirds were former, current or prospective forum members. This gave a different picture from the interviews with national voluntary organisations. Most survey respondents felt that support for forums could only be provided by an independent organisation outside the NHS and that NHS involvement would compromise the independence of forums. This presented some problems for the Department of Health who had been thinking of returning to the model of staff employed by the NHS and accountable directly to forums. One forum member, ex-CHC, summed up her view, which proved prophetic: '*forums have just signed their own death warrant!*' (Hogg, 2006p).

Without any clear answers about the way forward for forums, nothing then happened. There seemed to be no alternative but to rethink the whole package and abolish forums. In January 2006 the Department of Health set up an Expert Panel to make recommendations to the Minister. It was made up of experts outside the Department with Ed Mayo, Chief Executive of the National Consumer Council, as chair. Initially it was not intended to include patients' groups but it was then widened to include Harry Cayton, National

Director for Patients and the Public, as co-chair and representatives from patients' groups. The Expert Panel proposed a new approach putting patient and public involvement in the context of wider citizen engagement (DH, 2006b). Following this, it was announced that PPI forums would be abolished and replaced by 152 local involvement networks to be commissioned by local authorities (DH, 2006c). There was no formal consultation, since it was felt that there had already been two years of discussion and further delay would have meant that the opportunity to include the proposal in legislation and abolish Commission for Patient and Public Involvement would have been lost for another year. Local involvement networks are discussed in Chapter 10.

The House of Commons Health Committee concluded: '*The abolition of PPI [forums] seems to have been driven by the need to abolish CPPIH rather than any real need to start again*' (2007: 3).

What went wrong?

The ostensible reason for getting rid of CHCs was to start afresh with a less combative approach that puts patients at the heart of decision-making. Instead of modest one-stop shops costing about £23 million (excluding the establishing costs within regional offices) there came a range of new institutions, at a much greater cost. The initial vision in the *NHS Plan* was not implemented. Forums did not elect members onto trust boards and became pale under-resourced imitations of CHCs, often kept together by a core membership of ex-CHC members. The implementation, a tough challenge, was mismanaged largely because of the failure to learn from the experiences of CHCs or the voluntary sector. Furthermore the resources put into national and regional structures meant that forums were left with very limited resources. The Commission thus spent less money directly on 572 forums

---

Box 9.3   How the Commission spent its money

It had been intended that 75 percent of the Commission's finances would go to the forums after the first year's setting up costs. However, this was not achieved.[33] Resources were spent on the national offices, the Knowledge Management System and regional infrastructure.

In 2004–05, the first full year of operation, direct patient and public involvement costs were £18.1 million, 56 percent of total expenditure and below the annual expenditure on CHCs (£23 million).[34] For 2005–06 it was slightly reduced to £18 million and 55 percent of total expenditure.[35]

The overall cost of setting up the Commission and forums up to 2003–04 was £66.78 million.[36] Furthermore the estimated cost of redundancies for the 390 CHC staff was £12 million.[37]

Source: CPPIH.

than had been spent on 180 CHCs, in spite of the enhanced budget (see Box 9.3). With the thrust of recruitment to bring new people into the system, members needed more support, training and guidance which many FSOs were not able to provide.

The Department of Health in evidence to the Health Select Committee in 2007 gave several reasons for the abolition of forums. They argued that the current system was poor value for money and too bureaucratic. Forums had failed because they were not representative of their communities and did not reflect the changes in health services, such as the increasing diversity of providers, the greater emphasis on commissioning and primary care and the need to include social care within the arrangements for patient and public involvement (House of Commons Committee, 2007). However, other reasons for the failure are strikingly similar to the reasons that CHCs were seen to fail: lack of clarity about the role, performance management, accountability and legitimacy and the lack of government support.

Failure to learn from CHCs

The Commission and forums started out in a difficult climate. CHCs should have either been abolished cleanly or brought into the new system and the new system built around them, then CHCs would have been inside trying to make it work. Many of the problems the Commission faced were a result of the reluctance to learn from the experiences of CHCs or work with CHCs in their final year to help in recruitment and learn about the local area. Decisions made by the Commission to contract out staff support for forums made sense if it was accepted that there could be no transition with CHCs. However, the little research there has been on the effectiveness of CHCs had shown that it depended largely on the energy and commitment of its paid officers (Moon and Lupton, 1995; Hallas, 1976; Klein and Lewis, 1976). A core of experienced committed forum support staff never developed. Most were not, therefore, in a position to advise or support members and help them to contribute in the most helpful way. Staff were also on lower salaries with poorer job security than CHC staff.

There had not proved to be a large pool of untapped volunteers and national advertising is not how to encourage people from disadvantaged communities to put themselves forward. Recruitment activity that works most effectively is local and targeted outreach in partnership with voluntary organisations. It seems likely that recruitment to forums was poor, not just because of apathy but because there was little support and nurturing available for those who did join the forums and an attempt to exclude people with experience. While CPPIH struggled to recruit and retain 4000 volunteers for the forums, the National Institute for Health and Clinical Excellence was recruiting for its Citizens Council. It received 4000 applications and 35,000 expressions of interest. In their study of the NICE Citizens Council, Celia Davies and colleagues (2006) found that it was important to nurture and support those participating in order to get results that were useful.

Addressing performance management

The Commission failed to appreciate that the original impetus that led to its establishment had been the need for performance management for the new forums – the Holy Grail for CHCs in the 1990s. Forums had clearer and more restricted core tasks and the Commission had powers to set standards and review their performance, but were reluctant to do this. Choosing to contract out forum support accentuated inconsistencies between forums. Setting up a three tier system – regional offices, FSOs and forums – put the Commission into a position where they could only communicate with forums through the FSO. This distanced and isolated them from forums, contributing to the deterioration of relations. The Commission failed to make itself indispensable to the Department of Health and the decision to outsource the support made it easier to abolish the Commission and forums.

The verdict on CPPIH by a regional manager was that: '*There was no bad intent, but senior management was misguided and naive. From the start it was set up in a way that set people against each other. The chair against the chief executive, the commissioners against the executive team, regions against the forum support organisations, forum support organisations against members and everyone against the Department of Health*' (Hogg, 2006l).

What were forums for?

There were also more underlying reasons for the failure – different understandings of what was wanted from user involvement. First, there was the confusion of the perspectives of patients and citizens. Rob Baggott (2005: 547) points to '*under conceptualisation of the relationship between consumerism and citizenship, a fault line that seems to run through many of the Blair government's public service initiatives*'. Unlike CHCs, forums were not to be political. NHS Trust forums were a consumerist approach to empowerment: set up to meet the needs of the services. Forums were attached to institutions, at a time where policies and practices were trying to break down the barriers between services and conceptualise in terms of the 'patient journey'. The structure was fragmented and members encouraged to look at health services, rather than wider community interests or public health, which were increasingly important following the Wanless Report in 2002 and *Choosing Health* in 2004. Patients with experience and understanding of living with cancer have an important contribution to make to improving services, but will not improve services for people with mental health problems. In fact they could distort management priorities because they may feel, based on their own experiences, that cancer services are more important than mental health services. PCT forums were community-based and had a broader remit which could have been more people-centred and concerned with rights and needs. However, members were recruited as individuals and lacked legitimacy.

Second, there is also an uneasy balance between representation and management. Tensions and confusion between roles of management and representation are recurrent themes in debates on patient and public involvement. Conservatives had been clear about the difference between management and representation in their early design for CHCs in 1972, but the incoming Labour Government did not see the issue as so clear-cut and gave CHCs additional powers and tasks which duplicated those of health authorities. This set up an ambiguity at the heart of the movement that had been a recurrent theme throughout the life of CHCs. The vision for patients' forums was for a body of people working with the NHS and supported by the PALS in the trust. The skills required for forums members were listening and com munication skills as well as in negotiation.

The *NHS Plan* proposed that each forum would have a representative on the trust board. Many were sceptical about how it could work (TAB, 2002b). The accountability of the non-executive directors is to the Secretary of State and they are responsible for meeting financial targets that are set for them. This is not compatible with accountability to the public and patients. Forums with only a few members and no lines of accountability could not give their nominated non-executive director legitimacy or credibility. Furthermore, the forum representative would have had to be appointed by the Appointments Commission and there would have been problems if the forum's chosen representative was not deemed suitable to become a non-executive director. The director appointed by the forum would also receive the same remuneration as other non-executive directors, which could cause divisions among members. This plan was never implemented.

Third, there were different views about the value to be given to 'independence' or 'partnership'. With people more willing to complain, clinical governance and external inspectorates such as the Healthcare Commission, an independent lay monitoring body, such as a CHC, is harder to justify. In the early plans forums were 'stitched' into the NHS, but amendments made them independent. A civil servant felt that the Commission in its advice to forums focussed on independence. '*Independence became all-important, more than working in partnership. They are more concerned about their independence even than CHCs. This was down to the Commission who kept stressing that forums were independent bodies. They did not ask people to join forums in order to help improve the health service, but stressed that it was about being independent inspectors with badges and rights whose job was to fault find*' (Hogg, 2006f). Ironically CHCs had been more 'stitched' into the NHS than forums proved to be.

Patient or community representatives, who are expected to be outsiders-inside, play two simultaneous roles. On one hand they need to face outwards to their communities and keep in touch with them and bring in their perspectives; on the other they are expected to be a critical friend to those providing or commissioning services. Not an easy task – particularly when an advocate for the interests of service users or local communities is closely linked to the managers of those services, they will have no credibility in their communities.

Lack of government support

Ministers had been persuaded in 2001 that it needed to replace some of the functions provided by ACHCEW, but times had moved on. It did not help

---

Box 9.4   Changes in the Department of Health

Between 2000 and 2006 there were three major reorganisations in the Department of Health.

Following the Griffiths report in 1983 managers became key players in health politics for the first time. In 1989 the NHS Management Executive was set up to deal with operational issues and was staffed mainly by managers from the NHS and private sector. The civil servants in the Department of Health maintained responsibility for policy, but managers from the private sector and the NHS seemed to offer more relevant skills to the NHS than the traditional civil service.

Policy and executive functions merged again in 2000. However, by this time the Department of Health had been transformed from an ordinary part of Whitehall to being a Department dominated by the NHS. By 2006 only five civil servants in the top 32 posts had been there more than five years and all but one had come to the civil service from the NHS or private sector. Traditional civil servants had provided stability and consistency. They were politically neutral and the machinery of government could run smoothly independently of the politicians who came and went. They talked to colleagues in other government departments and so were able to avoid some fragmented or ill-thought through government policies.

Between 2000 and 2006 there were staff cuts. High staff turnover meant that there was a poor organisational memory and poorer understanding of the complexity of the NHS and the politics of health. By 2005 there was only one career civil servant among the 32 senior managers in the Department of Health.

Source: Greer and Jarman, 2007.

---

that four Ministers were responsible for patient and public involvement among their many other responsibilities between 2000 and 2003 – Gisela Stuart, Hazel Blears, David Lammy and Rosie Winterton. There were also three major reorganisations in the Department of Health between 2000 and 2006. Ministers increasingly looked for advice from their political advisers, whose main interest was the political standing of their minister. Greer and Jarman (2007: 26) conclude: '*As with many problems in the civil service, the problems here are ultimately with the ministers. If politics demands a department geared to centrally managing the English NHS, and often managing it very badly, then the civil service will provide such a department*'. The changes in the Department of Health are summarised in Box 9.4.

Legitimacy and accountability

The legitimacy and accountability of forums and the Commission were not addressed in framing the legislation. There was no agreement between the Commission, FSOs or forum members themselves about accountability or how members acquired their legitimacy. Forum members were appointed as individuals and did not necessarily have any links to others in the community. Forums had many fewer members than CHCs and no co-opted members.

Forums were expected to act as a conduit for local views rather than represent their own views. This required contacts with and the confidence of local communities. Though they were expected to be a channel and link with local communities, they did not have the staff support or resources to do this effectively. Like CHCs, forums were expected to represent people from disadvantaged communities or whose voices are not heard. Many CHCs attempted to involve people from minority ethnic communities as members and in their activities, with mixed success. CHC members were accused of being white, middle class and middle-aged (Cooper et al., 1996). This failure on the part of CHCs, though their record was probably no worse and sometimes better than other agencies, was one of the criticisms used to justify their abolition.

Forums like CHCs before them were criticised for being unrepresentative. This accusation is difficult to counter since no group can be representative. By the nature of their appointment they are unrepresentative. The actions of the group are more important than its composition: whether it can find ways to get to hard-to-reach groups.[38] CPPIH was successful in attracting new people, with one-third of members who had not volunteered before and one-third who had volunteered before but not in health, ten percent were from ethnic minorities. There was less success with age. Fifty-five percent of forum members were over 65, and only ten percent under 45.[39] CHC members were more diverse than forums members, with more women and more younger people. Younger people employed by voluntary organisations were elected as members, and members had support and contacts in the community to encourage them to continue. The regional appointments to CHCs were used to fill any gaps. The exclusion of voluntary and community groups from forum membership led to isolated individuals with no natural constituencies to which to report.

Conclusions

As the tale unfolds it is easy to see how things might have been done differently and might have had a different outcome. Involving users and citizens is more complex than government and the Commission anticipated. Unless there is respect for the people who you want to involve and the basic principles of openness and transparency are observed, it is likely to fail regardless of resources. The ill-fated Commission for Patient and Public Involvement was a costly failure in resources, public goodwill and credibility. The Commission itself had complex and unclear accountability to ministers and forums. Decisions that fundamentally affected many people were made in secrecy without consultation – the decision to abolish CHCs, the decision to contract out forum support to external organisations, the decision to abolish the Commission and then forums themselves. These decisions seem to have been made without an understanding of the likely implications. The lack of openness and transparency led to poor decision-making. The organisational memory and experiences of CHCs and much of the voluntary sector were ignored.

Following the announcement of the abolition the debate moved on to citizen engagement and integrating 'voices' in health and social care. Political commentators, such as the Power Inquiry, were also pointing to the fundamental lack of democratic accountability in the way that government and quangos like the Commission act. This is discussed in Chapter 10.

Renewing Democracy

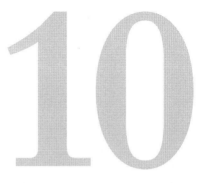

'Go to the people, live amongst them, start with what they have, build with them and when the deed is done, the mission accomplished, of the best leadership, the people will say "we have done it ourselves"'. Lao Tze (600 BC).

Overview

This chapter looks at developments since 1997 that attempt to address issues of citizen engagement.

- Decisions are being devolved to local level and neighbourhoods as part of democratic renewal.
- There are new ways of involving patients and the public in the NHS through members of foundation trusts, petitions and online surveys.
- Local involvement networks (LINks) replaced patients' forums in 2008, commissioned by local government.
- Each UK country has followed different models for patient and public involvement.
- All the initiatives described have increased the opportunities for participation, though there are questions as to whether it has increased citizens' ability to influence decisions.

Introduction

While media attention focussed on the bitter territorial battles between CHCs and the Commission for Patient and Public Involvement in Health (CPPIH), the action had moved to other arenas – promoting choice, health information and democratic renewal.

Policies in the 1980s had led to an increasingly divided society with high levels of unemployment, rising crime and antisocial behaviour. The reduction in social rights in the Thatcher years had meant that many members of society were not able to take part in the wider community. This had led to

149

the exclusion of large sections of British society, leaving people feeling powerless. This was seen as a major factor in the rise of crime and antisocial behaviour. When people become disengaged from representative politics, it is a threat to social cohesion, not just democracy (Faulks, 1998: 125).

The Labour Government when it came to power in 1997 wanted to address the problems arising from social exclusion and alienation and to re-establish public confidence in government. The independent Power Inquiry was set up by the Joseph Rowntree trusts to look into the problems of the disengagement of citizens in the political process. The Inquiry saw the problem as one of a deep political malaise where political institutions and politicians are seen as failing and disconnected from the great mass of the British people (Power Inquiry, 2006). The issue was no longer seen to be overcoming the democratic deficit in the NHS, but a more fundamental issue about the nature of representative democracy itself. Elected representatives in Parliament and local councils, held to account by the electorate, were no longer seen to be enough.

While responsibility for health policy was devolved in Wales and Scotland, in the early years of the Labour government power was centralised in order to try to push the NHS into 'modernisation'. However, this also centralised blame. By 2002 ministers became convinced that the answer was to decentralise and insulate themselves from political exposure on the day-to-day problems of the NHS. Decision-making was devolved downward within a national framework, including foundation trusts, practice-based commissioning, petitions and e-democracy. There were also devolution to local government who were now seen as community leaders. This provided opportunities for the closer links in user involvement in health and social care following the abolition of the CPPIH.

Foundations trusts

Even before patients' forums had been set up, the Government was looking at different ways of involving the public through foundation trusts. The inspiration for foundation trusts was mutual aid societies. Supporters came from the right and the left. Some in the Labour Party heralded foundation trusts as a new form of democracy and a rebuilding of popular socialism. Ian McCartney, an MP not generally considered a stalwart of New Labour, welcomed the idea, claiming: '*They lock the public resources of the hospital into ownership by the citizen in the community: owned by the community, for the community, serving the community*'.[1]

Foundation Trusts are a new type of organisation, known as public benefit corporations with a legal duty to provide NHS services to NHS patients. 'Ownership' is transferred from the Department of Health to the membership, which is drawn from people living in the localities served by the trust, patients, employees and local stakeholders, such as other trusts and universities. Members elect a board of governors. An independent regulator, known as Monitor, was set up to make sure they are well-managed and financially strong. Ministers no longer had to answer questions in Parliament about the operation of individual foundation trusts.

Membership

With no accountability to Parliament, governance arrangements become crucial. Individual patients and members of the public provide the basis for this accountability. The first trusts recruited between 1000 and 16,000 members in different ways, with different criteria for eligibility and different methods of organising elections (Healthcare Commission, 2005). Some trusts enlisted all patients and staff as members who could then opt out; others relied on people who were eligible to apply to join. Day and Klein (2005) found enormous variations in the number of members and their commitment, with the lowest membership in urban settings particularly in the North. By 2006 more than 500,000 people were members of foundation trusts. There is no minimum number of members and it is not clear what level of engagement is required to meet tests of community empowerment and democratic representation (Lewis et al., 2006). There is no requirement for members of foundation trusts to be representative or accountable. People will become members for very different reasons: some will join to promote better local healthcare. Others may join because they have strong views about abortion or to promote the needs of gays or lesbians or people from minority ethnic communities. All these are good reasons for joining as members, but could undermine the legitimacy of the trust if any group came to dominate. It is not easy to see how trusts can ensure a balanced membership of community interests and it is possible that they may need to introduce restrictions in membership to protect themselves from takeover by specific interest groups.

The board of governors is elected by members from constituencies of patients, public, staff and other stakeholders. The board must have a majority of members elected by the public constituency and, if there is one, the patients' constituency. Though the community and patient representatives have a built-in majority, their unpredictability, diversity and lack of experience and support mean that they may not work in a concerted way and so they may have limited power.

There has been confusion about the role of governors (Healthcare Commission, 2005; Lewis, 2005b). Was their role to provide community views to the board, help shape the corporate strategy of the hospital, provide independent scrutiny, act as ambassador to promote the work of the hospital to the community and other stakeholders or handle individual members' concerns? Day and Klein (2005: 28) questioned the role of governors and their accountability to local people. *'Elected governors are not responsible for the performance of their trust: they do not exercise direct control, have no right of veto and have only the nuclear option of sacking the chairman and executives... so elected governors can at best only hope to exert some influence. But how can anyone be held accountable for the exercise of something as intangible as "influence"?'*

It was not originally intended that foundation trusts would have forums, but concessions were made as the Bill went through Parliament. The Healthcare Commission (2005) reported that there was an overlap of function between the board of governors and PPI forums – both seeking to represent the public and patients and both competing for a limited number of volunteers from the same local community. The similarities of roles had, the Healthcare Commission concluded, caused confusion, conflict and duplication of effort.

Legitimacy and accountability

The legitimacy of foundation trusts has been questioned. Wilmot (2004) argues that, despite increased autonomy and responsibility, NHS organisations remain a part of the state healthcare system and are accountable to the Secretary of State. Though members ostensibly 'own' the trust, the trust is required to meet the mission of the Department of Health. The membership cannot change the purpose of the organisation and so are, in effect, there to carry out the purposes of the Department of Health.

In terms of democratic accountability foundation trusts are flawed. Allyson Pollock (2004) has argued that foundation trusts have restored powers to vested interests as arrangements for needs-based planning and fairness in resource allocation were dismantled. For example, there is no reason for foundation trusts to provide services to local areas or regions, if they do not find them profitable. The public as citizens need to be involved in planning and choosing priorities but this should be focussed on commissioning decisions, rather than service providers, such as foundation trusts. An independent working group for the King's Fund (2006) suggested that the 'voice' element – speaking out for the community – provided by the membership – should be removed from foundation trusts and placed solely with primary care trusts (PCTs) since they are the commissioners for their local community and the place where voices should be heard. NHS managers too felt that the duty to consult should be placed on commissioners, not providers.[2] Just as there was duplication between forums and foundation trust members, so there may be duplication between LINks.

Strengthening user involvement in primary care

National policy since the 1960s had tried to shift resources from the acute sector to primary care. But acute service providers have continued to dominate and consume a disproportionate share of resources. Public involvement in family health services is undeveloped. CHCs had no formal rights in relation to family health service practitioners. Close working relationships did not develop between GPs and CHCs (Hogg and Joule, 1994). The problem was not just that CHCs had no legal rights, but also the attitudes of many GP practices. GPs saw their accountability to patients as part of the doctor-patient relationship where there was no place for collective approaches.

Some enthusiastic GPs set up patient participation groups in the 1970s, but these groups were mainly supportive to the practice rather than challenging. They had limited impact and worked best where communication was already good between patients and doctors and did not develop in areas where they are most needed. Only about 3 percent of practices had established groups by the mid-1990s, but there has been an increase since 2004 (Pritchard, 1994; NAPP, 2007). There is a risk that practice-based groups might increase inequalities between patients. People who participate are likely to be older women in higher socio-economic classes and this may lead to policies that reduce access for some groups of patients. Some people, for example, may prefer not to share a waiting room with homeless people or people with drug or alcohol problems (Agass et al., 1991).

The lack of public involvement became more noticeable in the 1990s as GP fundholders started to decide which services to commission on behalf of their patients. However, little changed. Though there was much talk about involving patients and the public in primary care and NHS bodies have a duty to consult under Section 11 of the Health and Social Care Act 2001, the mechanisms for involvement were still fragmented and limited. PPI forums, set up in December 2003, were given rights in relation to primary care, but had not got to grips with this task before their abolition was announced. It seems that many GPs found it difficult to believe in the value of being responsive to patients or the public collectively or to commit themselves to formal consultation mechanisms. A study suggested that PCTs used patient and public involvement in their relationships with GPs as a way of controlling the medical profession rather than to promote the needs and preferences of citizens and users (Milewa et al., 2003). So far the main objectives seemed to be to deal with recalcitrant providers, rather than actually shifting power in decision-making.

The White Paper in 2006, *Our Health, Our Care, Our Say* promised a broader vision for general practice and primary care, incorporating community health and social care and giving more priority to preventive care. PCTs were expected to shift resources out of the acute hospital sector, in partnership with practice-based commissioners and local authorities. However, there was little emphasis on patient and public involvement and no real incentives for practices and clusters to carry out realistic and useful patient and public involvement (NHS Alliance, 2007). Commissioning decisions are complex. There is not enough money to fund all the services that users and professionals want so that managers need to balance the interests of some groups of users or some groups in the community against each other. The demands of articulate patients may actually increase rather than decrease inequalities.

Mass participation

Electronic technology presents possibilities of mass participation without taking up too much of people's time – through online surveys, mobile phone texting and petitions. Through these methods impressive numbers of people can be said to have 'participated'. However, the results may be more predictable and easier to control than deliberative processes. Surveys and opinion polls inevitably give simple answers that may reflect the way the question is asked and expect people to give a view on an issue they may never have thought about and in which they may have no interest. Referenda or online surveys give equal weight to everyone's views, however informed or uninformed. The results may be perverse – based on misunderstandings, incomplete or inaccurate information. People may react to a different question altogether. Voters, for example, may react to an unpopular government rather than to the issue on which their opinion is sought. These methods enable people to give their views on policy issues directly without needing to understand the issues or having their views mediated through elected representatives or other bodies such as CHCs or forums, which have an organisational memory.

The choice of technique determines the role that citizens are allocated and whether they are to be active or passive. It also determines how much autonomy managers themselves are prepared to give up. Participation initiated and managed by the NHS or local government tends to be limited and controlled and to focus on services rather than on reflecting what people want which may not fit so neatly into the way services are planned and delivered. Such methods do not contribute to an increased sense of community or social cohesion.

The critical issue in participation is who initiates it, who controls the process, what happens to the information and how it is used. They represent a move away from deliberative arrangements for citizen engagement. Deliberation takes time and requires reflection and weighing the evidence before coming to a decision. Without deliberation democratic choices are not exercised in a meaningful way.

E-consultations

In recent years the government has favoured market research techniques in their consultations. These were used in the consultation on the support

---

Box 10.1   Our Health, Our Care, Our Say

The consultation leading to the publication of *Our Health, Our Care, Our Say* was one of the largest and most ambitious public engagement exercises ever mounted in the UK.

In 2005 Opinion Leader Research ran four regional events around the country and 35,000 people answered an online survey, culminating in a national event attended by around 1000 people in October 2005.

An independent evaluation found that policy makers felt that the consultation had influenced the eventual White Paper and most participants felt very positive about being involved in the process. One weakness identified was that some participants wanted to stay involved, but there was no follow up.

The exercise was a success in terms of numbers involved, but more complex debates, such as about trade offs between different options and resource constraints, did not take place as had been hoped (Warburton, 2006). The total cost of the consultation was £1.24 million.[3]

Box 10.2   Democracy through the web

There are websites that encourage 'customers' to report problems and give feedback.

Neighbourhood Fix-It

This is a web-based mapping tool to make it easy for people to talk to their local authority and other local people about broken civic infrastructure in their neighbourhood. The website has been developed by mySociety and the Young Foundation, with funding from the Department of Constitutional Affairs Innovations Fund.

It aims to turn reporting faults from a private into a public experience where anyone can see what has been reported. It can include more people in the process of maintaining and improving the public infrastructure and environment in neighbourhoods.

Patient Opinion

This is a website where people can leave feedback about their local services. The inspiration is eBay, the online auction house, where control is through the feedback given by sellers and buyers. Through the feedback provided health services will acquire a 'reputation' and, it is hoped, that reputations will become an additional consumer power to exit and voice in the future.

Sources: http://www.fixmystreet.com, http://www.patientopinion.org.uk/

needed by forums when the abolition of Commission for Patient and Public Involvement in Health was announced and the consultation leading to the publication of *Our Health, Our Care, Our Say* (see Box 10.1). The internet can be a top-down method of communication but can also be used by citizens to regain control. It can be a way of circulating and highlighting information. The internet provides a chance for access to information and greater transparency and opportunities for those responsible for public service to answer questions broadcast live (see Box 10.2).

Petitions

The White Paper in 2006, *Our Health, Our Care, Our Say* promised that the public would be able to trigger reviews of local services. Where a specified number or proportion of people petitioned the service provider for improvements, the provider would have to respond, within a specified time, explaining how they would improve the service or why they could not do so (DH, 2006d). While the right to a response was heralded as new, but it was a right that CHCs had from 1974.

Petitions are most likely to be adopted by special interest or political groups and have limited value in making complex decisions since they favour causes or services that are popular or where users are well organised. Services, such as those for mental health, learning disabilities or older people, are likely to be ignored. For example, the implementation of NICE guidelines, such as access to drugs for multiple sclerosis (MS), is low compared to drugs for other conditions, such as breast cancer. At local level a petition to save the job of a MS nurse might be up against campaigns for local cancer services.[4] It would be up to the PCT or GP practice to decide if a petition was worthy of attention and, without additional resources, there is unlikely to be any significant change. There would also need to be arrangements for petitioners to appeal against the PCT's decision. The Scottish Parliament has been hearing petitions about major changes or service reviews since 1999. It has a public petitions committee to advise petitioners, hear their cases, take evidence and make recommendations for action by the Parliament. The appeals are about process. It cannot demand that a health board overturns a decision, but can ask it to demonstrate that it followed proper procedures. However, in the end petitioning rights were not included in the legislation. PCTs were given a new statutory duty to respond to local people, explaining the activities they are undertaking as a result of patient and public feedback on their services.

Emphasising petitioners' rights is another move away from deliberative processes. The only way to achieve some credibility and consensus will be through open and deliberative processes. Making decisions about the allocation of resources on the basis of petitions or judicial reviews of funding decisions is not the way to provide equitable services. Such decision can distort planning and decision-making and increase inequalities.

Local authorities as community leaders

While the NHS experimented with new forms of democratic participation, there were more radical changes with the modernisation of local government. The Local Government Act 2000 separated the executive from the representative role of councillors. Local authority overview and scrutiny committees (OSCs) replaced the committee system that had operated in local government for over 100 years. Councillors, who were not on the executive, now had the role of representing their constituents and monitoring the executive.

Double devolution was proposed, whereby government devolves decisions to local government who in turn devolve them to neighbourhoods. Devolving decisions in local government was seen as a part of democratic renewal. *Together We Can* was launched by the Home Office in 2005 as an interdepartmental action plan to strengthen citizens' engagement in delivering local services, covering health, schools, local authorities and the police. The Lyons Inquiry was set up in 2004 to consider the funding and functions of local government and its future role. Local government was to take responsibility for influencing things beyond their service responsibilities and become 'place shapers' and the voice of the whole community (Lyons, 2007). The Lyons Inquiry envisaged a more contractual approach between central and local government. Councils and their partners would have more control over their financing with less ring-fenced funding, less red tape and more flexibility in how they worked. Local area agreements provide the opportunity to create an agreed framework for service delivery and neighbourhood development. The White Paper, *Strong and Prosperous Communities*, gave a stronger role for health services in local area agreements by taking a lead in areas such as mental health with joint budgets and targets agreed at local level (DCLG, 2006). Like local authorities PCTs were encouraged to begin developing local area agreements (DH, 2006d).

People may be more likely to engage with services and policy-making at a neighbourhood level, especially in more disadvantaged neighbourhoods where their choices are more likely to be determined by their immediate surroundings (JRF, 1999). However, defining neighbourhoods is not straightforward, since there is often a discrepancy between administrative boundaries that are useful for efficiency and those that people relate to. Definitions of neighbourhood varied in local area agreements from areas with populations from 8000 to 60,000. The size of local government areas in the UK in relation to the population covered is large in comparison to other local government systems, at least four times as large as most other Western democracies (Stoker, 2005). Too much stress on neighbourhoods can lead to increased inequalities, as some neighbourhoods will be in a better position to influence decisions than others. The focus of double devolution is on a power rather than a poverty gap (Lepine and Sullivan, 2007).

The main way in which local people hold their local council to account is through electing councillors to represent them. Political parties in the twentieth century had an important role in mass democracy. There has been a substantial decline in the membership of political parties in the UK from over three million in the 1960s to around 800,000 in the 1990s. Forty years ago

---

Box 10.3   Loyalty to community or party?

In September 1998 Worcestershire Health Authority announced the downgrading of Kidderminster General Hospital by transferring the accident and emergency service, general medicine and surgical services to Worcester's new Royal Infirmary.

A local campaign group, Save Our Hospital, with Dr Richard Taylor as its chair, decided to fight the decision. The Council became involved in the campaign and councillors from all parties attended the marches and public meetings. The Health Authority's decision went to appeal to the Secretary of State who confirmed the downgrading, apparently supported by the local MP.

Once the decision had been confirmed by the national government, the Labour group felt no further action could or should be taken. From being seen by the local councillors as a legitimate campaign group, the Labour group began to describe the campaigners as extreme, inexperienced and biased. Local people were disillusioned by this. It seemed that they were criticised for being either uninterested or too interested in local affairs.

The campaign group, now called Health Concern, put up candidates in the local elections so that they became the controlling party on the council in 2002. Dr Richard Taylor stood for election to Parliament in 2001 and won. He retained his seat at the 2005 election.

Source: Crow, 2002.

44 percent of electors said they identified very strongly with a political party, in 2001 only 14 percent said the same (Power, 2006). Though political parties dominate the organisation of local, national and European elections, their connections with their local communities are weaker than ever before. Elected councillors can be torn between party loyalty and loyalty to their constituents (see Box 10.3). Reduced membership means that political parties can no longer provide a strong base for local democracy. At present councillors, according the Lyons Inquiry (2006: E40) are *'unrepresentative, poorly rewarded and undervalued'*. With the separation of the executive and representative roles of councilors, how they are held to account is less clear. Councillors, who are not on the executive, are now community workers rather than decision-makers (Chandler, 2001).

Restricting councillors in practice to nominees from political parties excludes many local activists and community leaders. There is likely to be a growth of non-partisan politics that will challenge local councillors as community leaders. Stoker (2005) suggests that there might be a role for the voluntary sector in this. They might provide the focus for single issue and non-partisan forms of political involvement and mobilisation.

Local involvement networks – Groundhog day?

In July 2006 the Department of Health announced that PPI forums would be replaced by 150 LINks. Debates started again about whether new local organisations were needed to mediate between the NHS and the public, apparently recreating CHCs. The Conservative Party proposed in 2006 new independent local statutory bodies called HealthWatch.[5] The British Medical Association suggested that the failure of NHS reforms since 2000 was due to the failure to engage the public. *'Given the scale of change there has never been a more important time to have effective patient and public involvement in the NHS, without which reform will be derailed. Without a real change in emphasis, discussion of reform is likely to be dominated by inflammatory and banner-based "debate"'* (BMA, 2007: 27). It recommended the *'formation of local health councils to provide a link between the community and health professionals/managers who are shaping local services'* (BMA, 2007: 19). Local health councils might be co-terminous with local authorities and provide a link between OSCs and the local community.

Initially the model for LINks was for a network which would *'act as little more than a conduit to enable health service organisations to contact a wide range of communities'* (House of Commons Committee, 2007: 4). This seemed similar to the public partnership forums which replaced local health councils in Scotland or CPPIH's vision for *'Our Health'*. They could be a resource available to trusts when they wanted to reach out to the community.[6] The problem with a network is that there is no core. Thousands can be signed up but their involvement may be limited and most could not receive training or support. This focusses on broadening the process of involvement rather than refining the outcome. It provides limited opportunities for informed deliberative debate. As a witness observed to the House of Commons Select Committee: '*If a smaller group of people can achieve something that everyone wants, I am not quite sure why we need everybody to be involved in the process*'.[7]

However, the model for LINks evolved beyond a network into a body more similar to CHCs than forums (see Box 10.4). In the Local Government and Public Involvement Act 2007 LINks replaced patients' forums. Like CHCs they were to be based on localities rather than institutions but cover both health and social care. They would focus their attention on the commissioning rather than the provision of services – a role that governments had been trying to persuade CHCs to do with little success since 1990. Otherwise they bear a striking similarity to the aspirations for CHCs and forums. LINks will, according to the Department of Health, aim to represent everyone in the community – not just existing activists but also those not currently being heard; have the power to investigate issues of concern; demand information, enter and view services, make reports and recommendations and refer issues to local councillors; and provide a one-stop-shop for to the community to engage with professionals and vice versa.[8]

Funding is provided by the Department of Health to local authorities to commission a 'host organisation' to develop the LINk, including recruiting members and developing and managing the governance structure (DH, 2006c). The use of external providers to 'host' the LINks is part of a wider policy to encourage the NHS to contract external support for commissioning.

Box 10.4   The Local Government and Public Involvement Act 2007

Each Local authority with social services responsibilities will have a duty to make contractual arrangements to ensure there are means for LINks activities to be carried out.

LINks activities will be:

• promoting and supporting people's involvement in the commissioning, provision and scrutiny of health and social care; enabling people to monitor and review the commissioning and provision of health and social care;

• Obtaining people's views about their needs for and their experience of health and social care; and

• Presenting people's views to those responsible for health and social care as well as making reports and recommendations on how services can be improved.

LINks will be able to refer matters to the OSC and receive a response.

Regulations impose duties on commissioners and some providers to respond to requests for information and to reports and recommendations made to them by the LINks; and allow entry by LINks to premises under certain conditions.

Source: Warburton, 2006.

One area specifically mentioned was patient and public engagement (DH, 2007b).

In spite of the political difficulties and the damaging loss of public goodwill following the abolition of CHCs, the Department of Health once again preferred to go back to the drawing board. The House of Commons Health Select Committee could not understand why forums should not be allowed to evolve. They advocated merging existing forums with LINks which would be less disruptive to volunteers and reduce the risk of large numbers leaving. Forum support organisations could have evolved into host organisations for the new LINks. The report concluded that: '*once again the Department of Health has embarked on structural reform with inadequate consideration of the disruption it causes*' (House of Commons, 2007: 3).

LINks offer greater opportunities to integrate participation in health and social care with wider citizen engagement. The Act gave few details about how they were to be set up, governance arrangements or how they would work (see Box 10.5). Those were left to secondary legislation and local decision-making. It was not at all clear how they will relate to practice-based commissioners or members of foundation trusts. There are four factors critical to the success of LINks: its powers, independence and accountability and whether it enables people to be engaged in ways they want. Particularly important is how the stability of LINks can be assured. They may not deliver what the government wants now and what the government wants may well change in the future. The terms on which LINks are established and how funding is provided will be critical for stability and public credibility.

Rights and duties

Without explicit rights there is a danger that either the LINk will be ignored by the community or may feel that the only way it can assert itself is by confrontation with the NHS or local authority and through the media, rather than working in partnership. People soon become disenchanted if they do not see any results or impact from taking part. However, in the real world consultation does not necessarily result in change, particularly where NHS bodies are driven by the market, prescriptive national standards and the need to keep within budget.

The main role envisaged for LINks is around commissioning services. Initially it was not intended that LINks would have any visiting rights to places where NHS services were provided. If LINks are about citizen engagement, visiting as mini-inspectors is not key to their role and duplicates the role of foundation trust members in the NHS. Rights to visit NHS premises were conceded in the publication of the Local Government and Public Involvement Bill, when it was clear that there would be opposition to the proposal otherwise. This right is limited to authorised representatives of the LINks and no visiting rights have been given for children homes and social care facilities that are private homes and visits might intrude on people's privacy. This excludes scrutiny for the most vulnerable people.

Box 10.5   Comparison of arrangements for patient and public involvement in England

	Community Health Councils 1974–2003	Patient and public involvement forums 2003–08	LINks (Local Involvement Networks) 2008
Number	182	572	150
Establishing body	Regional NHS office	CPPIH	Local authority
Coverage	Locality based	All NHS trusts and primary care trusts	Local authority
Remit	NHS, including public health	NHS, including public health	Health and social care
Number of locally members	15–25	Minimum of seven	To be decided
How members appointed	½ by local authorities, CPPIH ⅓ elected by voluntary sector, remainder by NHS regions	By application to organisation	By local host
How accountable	Not clear, but locally nominating organisations had power to remove members	To CPPIH	To be decided
Staff	Staff selected by members and employedby the NHS	Staff employed through voluntary organisations contracted to provide support	Staff employed by I host organisation
Access and premises	Local office in each district	No local offices	Local host organisation
Rights and powers	Rights to information, visits NHS premises, observer status on Health authority boards, to be consulted on major changes and appeal to the Secretary of State	Rights to information and visit NHS premises	Right to refer matters to the OSC and receive a response

Source: Hogg, 2007d.

LINks have few rights in relation to planning and commissioning of services. LINks have the right to refer concerns to the local authority's OSC. The OSC have an obligation to consider the referral and decide whether or not to take up the issue. In reality this means that any influence the LINk has will depend on the relationship it has with the OSC. As LINks have few statutory rights, it will be up to the Healthcare Commission and its inspection powers to ensure the NHS works with the new bodies. But this will not address the way that local authorities play their role as the 'establishing body' or themselves relate to the LINk.

Independence and accountability

Important for the credibility of the LINks will be whether the public see them as independent. State sponsored participation is always open to the accusation that it is manipulation – a cynical attempt to get support for management rather than enhance participatory democracy (Cooke and Kothari, 2001). The new networks will be hosted by a local organisation commissioned by the local authority. It had been intended that NHS bodies might host the LINks, but this was overturned in the House of Lords, thanks to a campaign by the newly formed National Association of Patients Forums.[9]

Accountability is not clear for LINks. While the 'host organisation' will be accountable to the local authority for delivering the contract, neither the local authority or the host will have any control of the LINks and governance will be a matter for the LINks membership (DH, 2007b). If a LINk was dysfunctional, the host would be powerless to change it and the local authority would only be able to hold the host organisation to account.[10] There is a potential conflict in that the LINk will be commenting on the services provided by the local authority. Furthermore local authorities vary in their support for the voluntary sector and some areas do not have co-ordinating councils for voluntary service. Control of LINks staff and budgets by members is essential for independence. The accountability of the LINks to their local communities needs to be explicit from the start and mechanisms set up to ensure transparency, including meetings held in public and annual reports.

LINks receive public funding and need monitoring to ensure that they do what they are supposed to and meet standards of probity. While CHCs and forums were criticised for their inconsistencies, LINks are expected to be different in each local area. Inconsistency, rather than a weakness, is now seen as a strength that demonstrates responsiveness to the locality. LINks require clear terms of reference, standards and arrangements for review, and lines of accountability and methods of reporting back to the community to which the network relates.

Terms of engagement

Will LINks be attractive or credible to the public and enable people to be engaged in ways that they want? A critical issue for health and social care in the next decade will be about eligibility for services and treatments. LINks may be expected to provide a way of determining local priorities for services – rationing by another name. Other forms of engagement – campaigning or petitioning – create barriers to rational and equitable planning and make PCTs vulnerable to pressure from interest groups that may not promote public health or the most effective use of resources. Deliberative processes enable possibilities for debate on priorities and an organisation, such as LINks, may be seen to be a vehicle for this. CHCs, acting as a mediating organisation, supported some but not all pressure groups. Sometimes this role could be abused, but CHCs could also ensure that counterbalancing arguments were heard from those groups which were not well organised or did not attract public or media support.

Most CHCs were unwilling to engage explicitly in the debates on rationing, and LINks may be no more enthusiastic for this thankless task. Commissioning, which is a complex and harder task to grapple with than commenting on provider services and results are likely to only emerge in the longer-term.[11] LINks need to operate in the public interest rather than the 'patient' or 'consumer' interest and this might lead to conflict since the major pressures for new drugs and new services come from patients and patients' groups, sometimes funded by the pharmaceutical industry. This raises the question of what kind of public health expertise is available to LINks.

Can local networks contribute to an increase in local democracy? For democracy to work at a local level there must be a variety of organisations so that citizens have many different opportunities to be involved in decisions about services. The NHS has always followed a separate path from local government, perhaps partly because it was looking to individual 'consumers' to drive change and promote the market in healthcare, whereas active citizenship arose from concerns about the anti-social behaviour arising from alienation in disadvantaged urban communities. LINks are based on local authority boundaries which may make relationships and collaboration easier. LINks could act as a platform to gather together people with interests in particular issues or localities in all aspects of health encompassing health, social care, housing and the environment are. With all public bodies having a duty to consult there is a danger of overlap, duplication and 'consultation fatigue' among the voluntary sector. There are therefore opportunities to take a wider view of citizen engagement, looking at services that have implications for health run by local authorities as well as the NHS.

Sustainability

There is also the question of the stability of the system. Some LINks will work well and some will not. Without ring-fenced funding, some local authorities, who already fund user networks, may feel that this is something they already do and LINks may become nominal. Contracts for host organisations were given initially for three years to 2011. The NHS Centre for Involvement based in Warwick University's remit is to work with the NHS staff to help them engage with patients and the public more effectively and support LINks (Tritter and Brittain, 2006). The Centre has a contract until

2011. The general policy directions suggest that LINks may once again be reformed to be more aligned to OSCs as providers of local intelligence.

Devolution and difference

Meanwhile there were changes in the other UK countries, with devolution the Scottish Parliament and the National Assembly in Wales were set up. All four countries inherited the same concerns about cost escalation, increasing patient expectations and demand, quality and value for money but each country has taken a different path, with different goals, ethics and under-standing of policy (Greer, 2004b). With the divergence in NHS policies in England, Scotland, Wales and Northern Ireland, there are opportunities to compare the different approaches (Box 10.6). There will be different lessons to learn from each country.

Wales

The NHS Plan for England had focussed on organisation, funding and the market. Wales focussed on localism and health outcome and chose to reform CHCs. When the announcement was made to abolish CHCs in England, the Department of Health had failed to warn the Welsh Assembly Government. From the start Wales was determined to keep CHCs and reform them. There was a consultation on future options for patient and public involvement, including CHCs. Most striking about the feedback from this consultation was the strong and consistent support for retaining and strengthening CHCs.

CHCs were reformed in Wales with little change to the basic model. They retained the dual focus on planning services and monitoring providers, working closely with the Welsh Assembly Government. For example, CHCs were funded to undertake the annual hospital patient environment visits. Complaints advocacy became a statutory duty with separate funding. There were changes in membership, with local authority nominations reduced from a half to one quarter, voluntary organisations members from one-third to one quarter. Half the members are public appointments are made by the Minister, The CHC chief officer and chair meet applicants and are involved in the assessment. These changes have made CHC more open with a more diverse membership, with more younger people than before. Some members receive payments for loss of earnings and carers allowances.

The Board of Community Health Councils in Wales was set up in 2003 as the establishing body for CHCs with delegated powers from the Welsh Assembly Government. All CHCs are represented on the Board which has 28 members. Both members and chief officers are full members of the Board, though there must be a majority of CHC members. The Board allocates budgets to CHCs, carries out performance appraisal of chief officers, oversees the annual CHC review process and appoints staff in consultation with the CHC. It provides a forum for CHCs to exchange information and undertakes training for staff and members, including a three-day induction for new

Box 10.6 Comparison of arrangements for patient and public involvement in the UK

	England	Northern Ireland	Scotland
Previous arrangements			
National	ACHCEW to 2003 CPPIH and PPI forums to 2008	No formal arrangements	Scottish Association of Health councils
Local	Community health councils to 2003 PPI forums to 2008	District committees to 1991 Health and social care councils (HSCCs) from 1991	Local health councils (number reduced to 15 from 34 in 1993)
New national arrangements	<u>NHS Centre for involvement</u> • Promoting user involvement in the NHS <u>National Voices</u> • Representing views at national level	<u>Patient and Client Council</u> Proposed in 2007 • Co-ordinating local involvement • Promoting user involvement • Representing views at national level • Promoting dialogue with public on health issues	<u>Scottish Health Council (SHC)</u> • Promoting and monitoring involvement carried out by health boards, and • Supporting improvement against agreed targets <u>Voluntary Health Scotland</u> • Promoting better links between the NHS and voluntary sector
New local arrangements	Local involvement networks (LINks) Overview and scrutiny committees (OSCs)	Proposed increase HSCCs from 4 to 5, co-ordinated by the Patient and Client Council	Public partnership forums Local Advisory committees of Scottish Health Council

Box 10.6 Comparison of arrangements for patient and public involvement in the UK – continued

	England	Northern Ireland	Scotland
Remit	Health and social care	Health and social care	Health care
Functions			
Consultation and planning	LINks OSC	HSCCs	Public partnership forums
Monitoring/inspection services	LINks – not main function but limited visiting rights	HSCCs	
Monitoring local involvement	LINks	HSCCs	Local advisory councils of Scottish Health Council
Complaints advocacy	ICAS contracted from voluntary sector by Department of Health	HSCCs staff	Independent Advice and Support Services contracted by health boards and provided by Citizens Advice Scotland through local CABx
Information and support to patients	Patient advice and liaison service (PALS) in the NHS	HSCCs staff	None
Management			
Involvement of patients and public	Individuals and organisations as members of LINks	Members of HSCCs	Individuals and organisations as members of public partnership forums Members of local SHC advisory committees

Box 10.6 Comparison of arrangements for patient and public involvement in the UK – *continued*

	England	Northern Ireland	Scotland
Staffing	Provided by host organisation commissioned by local authority	Appointed by HSCCs, employed by NHS Proposal that staff may in future be employed by Patient and Client Council	Provided by community health partnership (NHS)
Performance management	Unclear	Unclear for HSCCs Proposed that a role for the Patient and Client Council	
Accountability	Unclear lines with local authority and host organisation	Unclear for HSCCs Proposed role for the Patient and Client Council	Public Partnership Forums to Community Health Partnership Local Advisory Committees to SHC.
Independence	In terms of NHS but not social care	Yes	No

members. In addition it co-ordinates responses to national consultations and collates information about patients' concerns across Wales and reports to the Minister for Health and Social Services in the Welsh Assembly Government.

The process of reform has been slow, with a few CHCs fighting to retain their autonomy. In 2007 the Board's Director was made the line manager for chief officers. Initially the Board did not have any powers to performance manage CHCs, the Welsh Assembly government asked CHCs to accept this of their own volition. Enforcing this would require a change in legislation. Robust arrangements for performance management was important to ensure that the charge of inconsistency, so often used against CHCs, could be tackled and the Board could collect evidence for the effectiveness of CHCs, essential for their long-term survival. For the moment CHCs are safe, enjoying cross party support. There may be moves in future to bring health and social care together and develop them as part of wider structures for citizen engagement. CHCs hope by then they will have the evidence to demonstrate the benefit of their activities.

Scotland

In 2000 with *Our National Health* Scotland abandoned the market and moved away from contracting in primary care, giving responsibility for planning and decision-making to 15 health boards. Patients replaced consumers once again. With the Scottish Parliament there were new opportunities for campaigning at national and local levels. Before devolution there were only three ministers in the Scottish Office and health was a very small part of their portfolio. After devolution ministers were available five days a week instead of half a day on a Monday. Local health councils – the Scottish equivalent bodies to CHCs – had new opportunities for lobbying Members of the Scottish Parliament (MSPs). At national level the Health and Community Care Committee provided opportunities for lobbying as never before for the Scottish Association of Health Councils, which frequently gave evidence to the Committee. However, this new dawn was short lived.

Local health councils were seen generally as ineffective and variable. Unlike CHCs they were not independent since members were appointed by the board and, as one observer noted '*the boards tended to choose people who would go native and so they lost contact with the public*' (Hogg, 2007e). By 2000 local health councils (LHCs) were keen for reform and the Scottish Office committed itself to developing proposals to work with local health councils and the Scottish Consumer Council to develop new structures for public involvement (Scottish Executive, 2000). The patient focus and public involvement programme was developed to attempt to change the culture of the NHS in Scotland. The purpose of the programme was to try and rebuild trust between the NHS and the public through consensus and more transparent decision-making. NHS Scotland was given a duty to consult the public and it was concluded that there was no longer a need for mediating organisations, such as local health councils (Scottish Executive, 2003).

In 2004 15 local health councils were abolished and a new organisation, the Scottish Health Council (SHC) was established with local offices in each of the 15 territorial health boards. The SHC is a committee of NHS Quality Improvement Scotland, which was established in 2003 to improve the quality of healthcare in Scotland, a role similar to the Healthcare Commission in England. The Council has its own chair and national council members and promotes patient and public involvement and assesses the performance of NHS Boards on the Patient Focus and Public Involvement agenda against a range of performance indicators. Each year the SHC agrees actions with health boards that will enable them to demonstrate improvement and provides them with support. The SHC's annual assessment and reports on major service change are submitted to the Cabinet Secretary for Health and Wellbeing. The SHC works on a 'no surprises' basis but if the Council feels that a consultation on a major service change has not been properly carried out, the Cabinet Secretary may not approve the change. In disputes ministers have backed the SHC.

In each NHS board area lay members are appointed to serve as voluntary members on a local advisory council for the SHC. This was largely a political decision, driven by the need to show continuity with local health councils. However, the role of local volunteers was different: to monitor the process of involvement, not to take part in debates about service issues. In practice this proved a difficult and unsatisfactory role for unpaid volunteers to carry out.

The consultative functions performed by local health councils were replaced in 2003 by public partnership forums, which are networks of individuals and voluntary and community groups. They are set up and managed by the 38 community health partnerships, which are committees of the health boards and provide a focus for the integration between primary care and specialist services and with social care. Each forum is different but many are virtual networks with limited opportunities to meet and debate. Public partnership forums elect at least one of their members onto the community health partnership board. Research commissioned by the SHC paints a broadly positive picture of forums (FMR Research, 2008). One indicator on which boards will be assessed by the SHC is the quality and quantity of their population in the public partnership forum.

However, not everyone was happy with these changes. There were concerns from patient and consumer groups about the lack of independence and lack of dedicated staff (SCC, 2004). The local organisational memory that lay with LHCs was lost as well as the national voice with the abolition of the Association of Local Health Councils. The differences between the rural and urban areas in Scotland had meant that there was often no consensus view among health councils on national issues. Following abolition the Scottish Executive developed different ways of involving groups directly and a new umbrella group, Voluntary Health Scotland, was set up with funding from the Scottish Executive to encourage better links between NHS Scotland and voluntary organisations.

Northern Ireland

Health and social service councils, based on a similar model to CHCs, had been set up in 1991 to cover the four health boards and had replaced district committees which had been set up at the same time as CHCs. They covered both health and social care and 40 percent of members were local authority councillors. Following the return of devolved government there was a desire to engage the public more directly.

In 2007, as part of a wider health reform, it was planned that the councils would be replaced in 2008 by a new non-departmental public body – the Patient and Client Council for Northern Ireland. This body was to have functions similar to CPPIH in England: promoting patient and public involvement and good practice; representing the views of the public at national level and promoting a dialogue with the public to help them to understand issues about choice and priorities within limited resources. Board members were to be appointed by ministers, with local specialist teams to support public and community engagement locally and also to deal with complaints (DHSSPS, 2007). The original model proposed in Northern Ireland was to set up a professional community engagement service, getting away from lay membership. Another distinct difference was the function of the new Patient and Client Council to promote public debates about rationing and priority setting.

However, though the Minister recognised that there was a need for better co-ordination and a stronger regional voice for the four health and social care councils, he was not convinced that a single central body was appropriate or the exclusion of locally elected representatives.[12] Following consultation, new arrangements may be introduced in 2009.

The 'Third Sector'

The voluntary sector is often described as the cornerstone of civil society and makes an important contribution to democracy. Voluntary organisations are not looking for votes or to make profits, and so are more likely to be trusted by the public. People nowadays are likely to get involved in their communities through voluntary organisations, rather than political parties. In the 2005 general election 17 million registered voters did not vote, but 37 percent of people, who told the Power Inquiry that they did not vote in general elections, were members of, or actively involved, in a charity, community group, public body or campaigning organisation. They may see joining campaigning groups as a more effective way of influencing decisions than formal political processes.

Until the 1990s most voluntary organisations had seen their role as additional and complementary to publicly provided services. They were supported by grants from local authorities rather than contracts for services. These grants were affected by the cuts in local authority services that resulted from the rate capping and cuts imposed on local authorities by central government in the 1980s. Then they were encouraged to compete to provide public services in the market. The existing research evidence, mainly from the USA, tends to support the notion that not-for-profit providers offer higher quality care than the for-profit sector, with better survival rates, and better performance against quality measures (Lewis et al., 2006).This compelled voluntary organisations to adopt more formal and professional approaches to their work: the services of well-meaning but unskilled volunteers were increasingly unacceptable to the user, or too risky in a more litigious society (Blackmore, 2004). However, the voluntary sector cannot take over functions from the state that involve coercion or taking away benefits. The strength of the voluntary sector is that it is trusted by the public and this trust could be lost. The loss of trust could affect their ability to act as an advocate and undermine their role in enabling participation and involvement in decision-making.

The voluntary and not-for-profit sectors have grown in response to government policies to contract out public services. They are now identified as the 'Third Sector'. This comprises voluntary organisations, charities and not-for-profit companies or social enterprises. However, it is not always clear whether the Department of Health is looking for better managers of existing provision; more choice; innovation; reaching the hard to reach; building community capacity or user and carer-led services to help engage people in their own health. All worthy goals but amenable to different solutions.[13] These developments provide challenges to the voluntary sector, in particular the tensions between their advocacy (democratic) roles and their service provider (consumerist) role.

Social enterprises

There are shifts in traditional ways of working for voluntary organisations with the rise of social enterprises. These are organisations set up like businesses but with public or social good as their objective. The Department of Health sees social enterprises to be a future way to deliver services that had been directly provided by PCTs. PCTs could then concentrate on their commissioning role, while primary and community health services were delivered by a wider range of providers. New social enterprise organisations can support general practices to carry out practice-based commissioning or provide community health services (Lewis et al., 2006). Social enterprises can be 'mutuals', with members rather than shareholders. The members may be direct beneficiaries of the organisation (such as foundation trust members) or they may be other stakeholders, including staff or a small group of members whose job it is to represent the interests of the wider community. The benefits of mutuals are seen to be that they can give a greater say to frontline staff, formally engage patients and the public and enable them to hold managers to account and they create a renewed sense of community 'ownership' of health organisations (Lewis et al., 2006). The new enterprises will need to operate in a business-like way that may not be compatible with transparency and they may become disconnected from their roots in the co-operative movement. Collaboration and sharing of good practice may prove difficult in an increasingly commercial and contractual environment (Marks and Hunter, 2007).

There have been concerns that partnership with government at all levels could create and reinforce divisions in the voluntary community sector (Carrington, 2005).There is an increasing divide between a few big charities and small charities, which do not fit in with the grand plans for public services. Nearly 90 percent of charities generate less than 8 percent of the sector's income and their income is static or falling. Smaller charities may be more likely to be user-led, innovative and take risks and are the gateway to services for many people, particularly the most deprived and vulnerable groups.[14] There is a danger that they are likely to be increasingly dependent on pharmaceutical industry funding.

Advocacy

While the healthcare market gives the voluntary sector the potential for secure long-term funding for some activities, other activities are likely to be harder to fund and may be jeopardised. There is a danger that charities move away from their original objectives to take on new roles defined by others. Government was concerned, according to Nicholas Deakin, about the voluntary sector and: *'its incurable propensity to lobby and campaign and thereby disturb the judgments of politicians with emotional arguments insensitive to the economic realities and lead them to meddle with the sacred harmonies of the market'* (2005: 23). Advocacy was threatened, especially where it might involve criticising or questioning national or local policies and their implementation. The Compact between the voluntary and community sector and the Government was drawn up in 1998 to safeguard the independence of voluntary organisations to speak out of behalf of their members and users. But a National Council for Voluntary Organisations (NCVO) report indicated that many organisations did not have confidence in this (Blackmore, 2004).

Research with mental health service user groups found that some had lost funding as a result of campaigning (Barnes, 1999). Some voluntary organisations felt more exposed and less confident in speaking out in public. The market encouraged competing interest groups rather than collective action to bring about social change. CHCs felt that that their relationship with the voluntary sector changed and became more complex when voluntary organisations became providers. CHCs became an important outlet to enable voluntary groups to air concerns in a way that did not threaten their contracts (Cooper et al., 1996). Voluntary organisations were not engaged in the same way with patients' forums and this outlet was lost.

It may be that the larger organisations will choose to follow the route of professional leadership, involving users in a consumerist rather than democratic way. The legal structure of charities requires a few trustees to be responsible for providing services for beneficiaries, which is a model more suited to traditional charities than to organisations concerned with mutual aid or empowerment. Advocacy may increasingly come from single issue and fringe groups who use stunts to get publicity for their cause, whether throwing flour over MPs in Parliament or climbing the walls of Buckingham Palace. The media attention these activities attract encourages activists to see such actions as a short cut and an effective way of getting a case across.

The NCVO has argued that the aim of policy should be the transformation of public services rather than transfer from public ownership. The voluntary sector needs to be involved in identifying service need, as a result of gaps in service provision, or poorly designed or delivered services; helping to design solutions to meet a need; and delivering services (Blackmore, 2006). This complexity in the roles of the third sector was recognised in the third sector review launched in 2006 by the Treasury and the Cabinet Office as part of the Comprehensive Spending Review process. The review takes a long-term view of what is needed for the sector to thrive over the next ten years. It puts greater emphasis on the advocacy role and the role of the sector in helping local authorities engage with communities and build capacity as part of the modernisation of local government (HM Treasury and the Cabinet Office, 2007).

Alternative management approaches

Different managerial approaches are needed for different services in the public sector. The market may have benefits in providing some services but is not suited to others. Alford (1998) argues that there is an alternative to the market model of contracting out public services – co-production. This is the involvement of citizens, volunteers and clients in producing public services as well as consuming them. The client or service user can be active in advocating levels or types of services but also active in their delivery. In the late 1970s and early 1980s, co-production attracted almost as much interest as marketisation, but since then it has attracted little official interest. The major theories were established between 1977 and 1984 but implementation floundered as the theories were largely interpreted as providing services using volunteers – who were not considered to be a sufficiently reliable base on which to carry out public functions. By ignoring co-production with clients, governments have closed off an important management approach.

Many public services are appropriate to co-production. Recycling schemes depend on people making the effort. Getting unemployed people into work requires the co-operation of the job seeker. In health and social care the effectiveness of any treatment or care package depends on the co-operation of the individual and carers. Services for people with long-term conditions may be particularly appropriate to 'co-production' since they may be able to communicate better with users than professionals (Barker et al., 1997). This can be particularly useful where there are boundaries between professionals and users that make communication and trust difficult to establish, such as around mental health issues, homelessness, problem drug and alcohol use. This includes services working with communities or groups who find it difficult to access services, whether because of language, culture or disability. Users or people from those communities can act as a bridge. Many helplines, community outreach, supported housing, drop in centres, befriending schemes and advocacy programmes employ people who have themselves used services (see Box 10.7).

The barriers in most user-led schemes tend to come from the ambivalence of staff to the breakdown of the professional–user boundaries. In the USA there are more established user-led schemes, though divisions have arisen between those that work with professionals and those that prefer to maintain the separatism. Rose et al. (2002) conclude that ideological differences in the consumer movement may hamper the development of new services.

National voices

Though more decisions may be devolved to local level, there may be little scope for local preferences to actually change services. Local managers must work to financial targets and national standards. Central control remains through arms length bodies, such as the Monitor, the Healthcare Commission and NICE, in effect reducing public accountability at national level. Where so many decisions that affect local people are made centrally, local bodies may find it difficult to balance policy injunctions imposed from the centre against local views and priorities elicited through consultation (Newman et al., 2004). Many services that are delivered locally are considered to be outside the bounds of local deliberation.

As long as there is a national framework of regulation and standards setting, a strong national voice for patients and citizens is essential in formulating health polices. In comparison to professional and commercial interests, the user or public interest voice at national level is weak. The only sanction citizens have against government is public opinion and influencing voters. Commercial and professional interests have much stronger sanctions. Decision-making has become fragmented with decisions being made by different NHS bodies, rather than a civil service department which has made it harder for voluntary organisations to influence national decisions. This already weak voice is further weakened by the dependence of many voluntary organisations on government funding and the lack of co-ordination and co-operation within the voluntary sector (Hogg, 1999).

Since the abolition of CHCs and their national association there has been little questioning of broad national health policies from a user or public interest perspective. Following the abolition of CHCs in England and local health councils in Scotland, there was interest in looking at models from overseas. The Netherlands and Australia have co-ordinated arrangements for involving users at national level (Hogg and Graham, 2001; Hogg, 2007c) (see Box 10.8).

Box 10.8   National organisations – Australia and the Netherlands

Australia

The Consumers' Health Forum of Australia (CHF) was established in 1987 following a call from a group of voluntary organisations for a formal system of public participation to be built into the national health administration. CHF is a coalition of national, regional or local community and consumer groups. It mainly works at national level through its community representatives programme where it recruits, trains and supports individuals nominated by member organisations to represent consumer interests on national government and professional bodies. CHF does not join campaigns, but may contribute information to members' campaigns. It is pragmatic in the positions it takes and aims to continue to work as 'insiders' even when they are not in agreement with policy, seeing this as the best way to influence them. It is funded by federal government.

The Netherlands

The Federation of Patient and Consumer Organizations in the Netherlands (NPCF) was established in 1992. It has 27 member organisations who themselves represent national umbrella groups. It is funded by government and is much better resourced than the CHF (with 35 full time staff compared to eight in CHF). Over the last five years the work of NPCF has mainly revolved around the major health reforms which were introduced in 2006. Before that NPCF had been involved in campaigning for legislation on patients' rights, including legislation on complaints, quality standards, medical treatment and consent, and the participation of clients in long-term care. Members are involved on national committees and councils in addition to projects. Recently they have extended their remit to provide health information to the public to help them act as consumers to encourage the development of the healthcare market.

   Though there are major differences between the UK, Australia and the Netherlands, in representing users' views at national level there are similar challenges and tensions. There are tensions between preserving their independence and receiving government funding. Both aim to work in partnership with governments and, within limits, they can be critical. However, retaining government funding leads to some explicit or implicit compromises in terms of advocacy. CHF does not campaign, while NPCF does lobby, but largely against vested interests with implicit or explicit government support. The perceived lack of willingness to speak out can lose the organisation credibility with members and cause tensions between members. However, being seen to be 'negative' by government is likely to lead to marginalisation and eventual loss of funding. This tension was evident even in the Netherlands where there is a tradition of using consensus to bring about change and the Government sees the importance of patients' groups in helping to undermine vested professional interests, which are more powerful than in the UK.

Source: Hogg, 2007.

There have been attempts to co-ordinate the views of voluntary organisations to give them a stronger voice in policy-making. The Patients Forum was set up in 1989 by the Patients Association, mainly as a forum for chief executives of national organisations to get together to comment on the implications of the introduction of the purchaser/provider split. It since focussed on information exchange and providing a platform for the Department of Health and other statutory and professional bodies to communicate with the voluntary sector, rather than co-ordinating and representing their views. The Long-term Conditions Alliance was set up in 1991 as an umbrella group for patients' groups. However, its focus is limited to long-term conditions and its acceptance of pharmaceutical funding has meant that some organisations, such as mental health organisations, do not belong.

There are difficulties in co-ordinating and developing a strong national voice for the voluntary sector. Some of the difficulties of co-operation within the voluntary sector are based on their origins, their relationship with professionals and how far users are involved in decision-making and governance. An organisation of disabled people, for example, is very different from an organisation for disabled people. Some may cover a very specific disease or condition and have limited objectives; others may represent the wider public or political interests. Researchers have identified different types of social movements in health (Brown and Zaestocki, 2004; Baggott et al., 2005). The most important distinction between groups, however, is related to governance or who makes decisions – whether the organisation is professionally dominated or user-led and its relationship with its funders. The second reason why co-operation may be difficult is that organisations are competing for the same funding sources and for the attention of the same decision-makers in campaigning to get priority for their issues.

One of the key challenges for umbrella organisations is how to keep the interest and commitment of members. Member organisations need to give priority to their own organisations and there will always be tensions between the views of different member organisations who have different objectives, attitudes and approaches to working with professionals and government. Whether or not to accept funding from the pharmaceutical industry is a divisive issue in all countries. In the long-term the different perspectives tend to lead to an increasing distance between members and the umbrella group. It also can mean that larger member organisations, with their own policy officers, lose interest and the umbrella organisation becomes less important for government. Smaller member organisations may remain in membership but they may have little capacity to be involved. This happened to the national voluntary organisation, the Patients Forum in England (Hogg et al., 2006). Some national campaigns have, however, been effective, such as the campaign against proposals for the reform of mental health legislation (see Box 10.9).

In 2006 in England ministers became concerned about the limited contacts between the voluntary sector and the government. The Department of Health funded a working group with representatives of the voluntary sector. This proposed the creation of 'National Voices' as a network of national not-for-profit organisations that would be *democratic, facilitative, supportive and powerful*' (Taggart, 2006; Taggart, 2007). National Voices is a charity, initially funded by the Department of Health. Starting work in 2008, the

> **Box 10.9   Campaigning on the reform of the Mental Health Act**
>
> In 1999 the Government published a Green Paper on the reform of the Mental Health Act 1983. Users and professionals were concerned about patient autonomy and discrimination, while the Government was more concerned with public safety and obtaining powers to force mentally ill people living in the community to take their medication and to detain those with severe personality disorders, even if they had not committed a crime.
>
> The Mental Health Alliance, a coalition of 80 organisations working together to secure better mental health legislation, included voluntary organisations, professionals and lawyers. After a consistent campaign by the Alliance, the Government dropped its more radical proposals in favour of amendments to the 1983 Act.
>
> *Source*: Mental Health Alliance http://www.mentalhealthalliance.org.uk accessed 24 April 2007.

main functions are to influence policy-making and enable two-way communications between members and the Department of Health. An advisory group of ten people drawn from member organisations would meet with Ministers every three to four months. It is not clear how LINks, which will be based in the voluntary sector, will be part of this new movement.

In Scotland the initial reason for exploring the need for a stronger voice at national level was concern in the Scottish Consumer Council about the difficulty in finding people able to represent public or patient interest at national or international levels and concerns about the effectiveness of existing representation (Hogg, 2007c).

Conclusions

There is no question about the national policy commitment in the UK to patient and public involvement and increased opportunities for participation. But is this democracy? The many new means of communication established between government, users, community groups and individuals may have given people less rather than more control over policy-making. There are inherent tensions between representative and participatory democracy. Participatory democracy sees the lines of accountability as multiple and overlapping. It involves a continuous exchange between the decision-makers and the public, with transparency, explanation and questioning. What do governments really want to achieve? Is it stronger accountability for public bodies or is it public consent for decisions and support for policies? Or is it about social cohesion and social inclusion? The English health reforms have been driven by marketisation rather than to strengthen civil society. Some initiatives described are aimed at inclusion and social cohesion and this is very different from participatory democracy. It has been argued that the real end product that the government aims for is a therapeutic one – enabling individuals to express their feelings, and feel that they are 'listened to' rather than to enable them to participate in decision-making (Chandler, 2001).

Participation is seen differently by those in power who invite participation and by those who are invited to participate. The interest at national level has been to develop and promote techniques for involving people, without giving them access to the more dangerous territory of the power relationship. Over the last 30 years participation has increasingly been seen as a tool of government and management and the power dynamics behind it overlooked. Sherri Arnstein looked at participation processes initiated by statutory authorities in the 1960s to improve the lot of poor people in urban ghettos in the USA and postulated a ladder of participation (Arnstein, 1969). Arnstein saw citizen participation to be about citizens' power. The bottom rungs of the ladder were what she describes as non-participation – therapy and manipulation, rising to citizen power, where there is partnership, delegated power and, finally, at the summit, citizen control (see Box 10.10).

Later commentators have accepted the continuum of participation, but have preferred to see the objective as about influencing decision-making rather than degrees of citizen power. Arnstein's ladder is seen as simplistic in that it confuses means and ends, implying that user empowerment should be the sole aim. It also fails to reflect the different forms of participation in health related decision-making. Tritter and McCallum (2006) argue that it is the process rather than the outcome that has the greatest potential for changing organisational culture. Concentrating on the power dimension takes little account of diversity and has the potential of reinforcing existing patterns of inequality. An empowering system needs to demonstrate safeguards to protect the rights of people with rare diseases, provide space for people with dissenting views, and those for whom services need to be tailored differently.

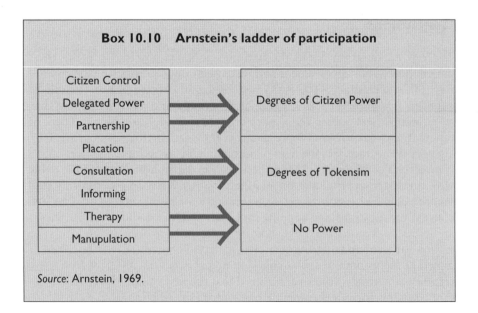

Box 10.10   Arnstein's ladder of participation

Citizen Control	
Delegated Power	Degrees of Citizen Power
Partnership	
Placation	
Consultation	Degrees of Tokensim
Informing	
Therapy	
Manupulation	No Power

Source: Arnstein, 1969.

Whatever the criticisms of Arnstein's ladder, it still provides an important insight into the core issues of participation which are about who manages the processes and the outcomes. Whether participation is managed by local government or the NHS, its contribution to participatory democracy is limited. There is a difference between autonomous citizens' groups that are brought together by their enthusiasm about some objective, such as a campaign around local services, and individuals brought together by the NHS or local councils to give them information or to consult them. Chandler (2001: 12) concludes this process feeds passivity and institutionalises an individual perspective rather than challenging it.

Chandler suggests that there may be more participation, but less democracy. The more democratic participation is seen as a tool of social policy, designed to address questions of social cohesion, the less likely it is that politically engaged citizens will emerge. He concludes that new forums and consultation groups promote democratic participation through little more than consciousness-raising and customer feedback. As a result, they *are more likely to institutionalise a network of passive individuals than create or empower active citizens*' (2001: 13).

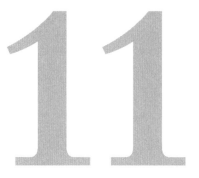

Conclusions

'Ever tried. Ever failed. No matter. Try again. Fail again. Fail better.'
Molloy, Samuel Beckett, 1951.

Overview

This chapter looks at what we have learnt from the last 30 years and what may happen in the future.

■ Containing the escalating costs of healthcare is the major concern of western societies.

■ The consumerist agenda will continue to be important but may increase inequalities and demand for health services.

■ Consensus on priorities and eligibility for healthcare may become more important for governments, and this too may increase inequalities as some groups come to dominate.

■ In extending participation the challenge is how to enable democratic engagement in these decisions without increasing inequalities and inequity in society.

■ Participation needs to be linked with equity and human rights can be a tool for empowering communities and addressing issues of discrimination and equity.

Introduction

The story of the last 30 years provides much to celebrate and much to mourn. Though the world has changed enormously since 1974, the issues that policy-makers tried to address in setting up CHCs are still current and seem to have advanced little. With all the rhetoric around patient and public involvement, it is easy to forget what the purpose of patient and public involvement is.

Why do governments want people to get involved? In the early days the main purpose was to curb the power of professionals, in particular doctors. Government used CHCs and voluntary organisations to help them implement national policies at local level, in particular addressing inequalities in the redistribution of resources from the acute hospitals to community and the under-resourced 'Cinderella' services. Then the interest moved to how patients as consumers could help shake up the system and create a market in healthcare. Choice and consumer rights were favoured over voice and collective approaches based on social rights. From the 1990s governments wanted CHCs to work with commissioners of services and become involved in setting priorities for services with them. CHCs were reluctant to get into this, seeing it as a management task or as a way of legitimising cuts. The *NHS Plan* abolished CHCs and set up systems to mainstream and diversify patient and public involvement, bringing representation closer to management, but this proved to go nowhere. In England LINks and membership of foundation trusts offered new opportunities.

However, even the questions about the processes remain unresolved. Should representation and management be separated? How do you achieve participation without interfering with the manager's ability to manage? Who do those who take part represent and how can they be held to account? Can users become 'insiders' and partners and still retain their independence and public credibility? What are realistic expectations of the benefits that engagement can achieve? Can the public help legitimise and achieve consensus on decisions about priorities? How do you motivate people to volunteer rather than relying on the 'usual suspects'?

Klein (2004: 207) observes *'the result of successive initiatives – each superimposed on previous ones – has arguably been to produce an incoherent system of public involvement'*. However committed one is to user involvement, it is tempting to agree that there has been an overinvestment in what passes for patient and public involvement in the NHS in England. User involvement is expensive in staff time and money, whether or not it is effective or appropriate. The problem with patient and public involvement for managers is that you do not necessarily get what you want from it and what you want can change. However you word the questions, you may get answers you do not want. You can, of course, then ask another group to get a different answer to support what you want to do. User involvement, like democracy, is complex and difficult and you can never get it right.

The views of patients and public are a minor part of the policy-making process. There is a discrepancy between the rhetoric of listening to patients and public and the reality of the power of patients and public. New Labour adopted the idea of evidence-based government. This involves integrating experience, expertise and judgement with the best available external evidence from systematic research. At present it is argued, policies are driven by values and resources. Instead they should be driven by evidence. The perceived advantage of evidence-based policy is that it replaces opinion-based policy and, as the evidence base increases with better research, opinion-based government will recede (Muir Gray, 2001). Involving people in decisions means listening to opinions which is not seen as a robust base for policy-making. Unfortunately patients and public only have opinions to offer. Qualitative research can provide 'evidence' but can still be seen as subjective. Opinions carry less weight than those of professionals or commercial interests.

In future there is likely to be less social cohesion and less consensus in society. With the global market and increased immigration, communities are becoming more diverse and it is harder to assess their needs. The UK is facing a rapidly changing environment, both domestically and internationally. There is a rapidly changing global economy in healthcare where patients have access to treatments and services in other countries and through the internet. There are more older people, living longer in poorer health who will make more demands on community and long-term services. Whatever happens there are likely to be changes in the way health and social services are delivered in England.

So far all the debates have been around how healthcare should be organised – the means, not the aims of the NHS. The NHS is based on a social contract where society agrees to pool resources and share risks that developed out of the shared experiences of the Second World War. It was set up as a national service funded by taxation to avoid inequalities in services depending on ability to pay and where you lived. For 50 years it has been a basis for social cohesion in the UK, however, this may not always be the case (Thornton, 2006). The USA is an example of a country where healthcare is not viewed as a social right for all its citizens.

In this book it has been argued that governments have attempted to shape user involvement to fit its policy concerns at the time. For what purposes will governments want user involvement in the future?

The consumerist agenda

The consumerist agenda will remain – to improve services to meet the needs of users, rather than providers, to improve access and take-up of services. The individual will have a continued role as the 'customer' who alone can report on how services met their expectations and needs and the sort of experiences they had. The individual is also likely to be expected to take more responsibility for their own health in return for the treatment and services they receive. It is not a long distance to begin to refuse treatment or limit services for those who do not abide by the 'contract'. People who smoke or are overweight might be refused surgery until they have stopped smoking or have lost weight. The evidence is that these policies will have most impact on people who are the most vulnerable and disadvantaged already.

There is likely to be a growing divide among people who know how to make the system work for them and those who do not; between the 'customers' that providers want to serve and those they wish to avoid, leading to an underclass of users. Many people feel themselves to be marginalised and want the support of their peers (Bolzan and Gale, 2002). Without support and advocacy for vulnerable groups, inequalities between individuals will increase.

It can be argued that in England there will soon no longer be a need for collective forms of engagement for people, patients and carers. The dream of managerialism of the 1980s of a health service run like Sainsbury's supermarkets might at last be fulfilled. The changes with payment by results where providers will be paid for individual patients will mean that there will be no need for additional incentives or sanctions for providers to satisfy their customers in a competitive market. In fact individuals may have their own budgets in future.[1] Rudolf Klein, an early researcher on CHCs, suggests that *'it is doubtful if the present system for patient and public involvement will be needed in its full, florid form'* (Klein, 2004: 211).

However, health is a more complex experience than this. Some 'consumers', such as mental health services users, want to redefine the identity that they have been ascribed by providers. With limited choice and sometimes unable to refuse services or 'exit', their rights as citizens are more important to them than their rights as consumers. The logical development of the self-care and expert patient programmes is for users to break out of this role and themselves become providers, offering a role model for others and breaking down boundaries between users and professionals. Such developments might be hampered by ideological divisions between the users who are separatists and want to do things alone and those that want to work with professionals. It is, however, the integration of users into many services working with equal status with professionals that has great possibilities for developing user-centred services.

Democratic engagement

The information from customer services is not sufficient to enable the planning of services. Some 'consumers' may want to work with staff to argue for more resources for the services they use and to gain priority over other services, potentially distorting rational planning. In terms of the public debate, they are only one of many voices that need to be heard. There is a wider role for individuals as citizens. Public involvement needs to be considered in a different, democratic agenda – with different purposes, methods and people involved. Consumerist and democratic approaches have been confused in national policy and patient participation has been seen as a proxy for citizen participation. CHCs and forums combined and sometimes confused both perspectives.

Devolving power to local level is leading to a greater convergence between the NHS and local government, and is highlighting the lack of democratic accountability for in the NHS. There is likely to be pressure for the democratisation of PCTs and the integration of NHS community services into local government (Thornton, 2006). By placing local involvement networks within local government, there is the coming together of several policies: attempts to increase social cohesion, the sense of belonging and 'Britishness'; to renew representative democracy; to integrate health and social care and to avoid difficult decisions and blame in Whitehall by devolving decisions to local level.

Increasing participation requires a variety of ways and levels so that people can be involved in the areas and the extent that they want. There will no doubt be an increase of e-democracy and online surveys which can involve large numbers of people. Many people may be willing to take part in online questionnaires or even attend an occasional meeting, but this is not enough to meet the requirements of informed decision-making or deliberative democracy. Complex decisions about healthcare and its resources need deliberation and informed debate that such techniques cannot provide.

What arrangements are needed to enable deliberation? The days of independent representative mediating bodies may to be over in most of the UK. CHCs, PPI forums and local health councils in Scotland have been abolished since 2000 and the future of health and social service councils in Northern Ireland is uncertain. CHCs in Wales are the only survivors. Mediating organisations that see themselves as the enabler of engagement, rather than acting as the gatekeeper, can still play an important role. CHCs at their best saw their role as agents for community development, supporting and encouraging smaller groups to get their views heard. Mediating organisations can also provide a useful buffer for voluntary organisations. Voluntary organisations dependent on the NHS or local government for contracts and funding may be reluctant to speak out on behalf of their users and it is easier to work through a mediating organisation.

The problem remains that people like the idea of participation, but may not have the time or enough interest to become actively involved. However, this needs to be addressed so that decisions made at local level are rooted democratically in communities. There will need to be an expansion in the pool of active citizens to take on these roles. Volunteering is a major part of maintaining a healthy civil society and social capital. Where will these volunteers come from? James Fishkin (1991: 57) believes that *'we have created a system that permits participation but has failed to motivate it effectively'*. Studies show that there are many benefits for the individual of volunteering, including benefits to self esteem and health (CSV, 2004).

The more that is required, the fewer people there are that are willing or able to get involved (May, 2005). Professionals and paid workers can be ambivalent about volunteers which means that volunteers do not feel valued or able to influence what is happening. The most engaged and most committed may be branded the 'usual suspects. Most people who get involved want to improve things and are motivated by experience; some are grateful and want to give something back, others are damaged and want change or even revenge. People who put themselves forward as volunteers can be awkward and obsessional. The involvement of those with experience should not block new people from getting involved but they can be mentors and trainers for new people who may need support to understand the complexity of the task of working in partnership in the planning of health services.

Unless the issue of motivating people to become involved is addressed, many LINks will be virtual organisations – a database of contacts that service providers can access. Unless you believe that you can make a difference or there is a financial incentive, there is no point in volunteering your time, especially if you are likely to be dismissed as a usual suspect! Members of CHCs, PPI forums and foundation trust governors received travel expenses only. The world was a very different place in 1974 when CHCs were set up. Then volunteers were involved in the NHS on health authorities and hospital boards as well as CHCs and did not receive or expect to receive payment. Now there are lay people involved in many capacities in the NHS and related statutory bodies, who receive substantial honoraria. This was not extended to members of PPI forums or foundation trusts which might indicate a lack of value put on their contribution. It also restricts who is able to take part. The Department of Health (2006e) has introduced guidelines on payment to users involved in the development and delivery of health services, suggesting that NHS organisations should have a payment policy for users and clear criteria for what they are expected to do for this.

Rationing and eligibility to health and social care

All Western health systems are realising that there are not the economic resources to meet the demands for health and social care indefinitely. Health and social care costs are rising and are likely to continue to rise. There are new medicines and treatments available as well as an aging population. Providing choice is itself expensive and requires an oversupply of health services. Individuals, often backed by the pharmaceutical industry, are using the High Court to seek treatment under the Human Rights Act for themselves or their groups, which their primary care trust may consider unaffordable or not cost-effective. NICE provides guidance on what drugs and treatments should be provided, but there is no guidance on what services should not be provided in order to fund new treatments.

Governments still act as if the problems of escalating costs can be solved by organisational change. Rationing decisions in the final analysis are decisions about who lives and who dies, who gets treatment and who does not. These debates raise ethical and political issues about what treatments society can or should afford to pay for. This leads to an unavoidable conflict between the individual's entitlement to healthcare and the state's responsibility to provide it.

These are decisions which no one wants to tackle. There is reluctance to raise a public debate nationally on how services should be provided and who should be eligible for free healthcare. In 2007 the British Medical Association (BMA) suggested that government must recognise that there will be rationing of services and that there will be an erosion of the standard of comprehensiveness (BMA, 2007). Only when society recognises that rationing is a reality can a mature debate develop that is open, equitable, and undertaken on the basis of social agreement. The BMA believes that Parliament is responsible for the financial decisions it makes about the scope and standards of services and should not devolve impossible tasks to the NHS. Decentralising decision-making as outlined in Chapter 10 may lead to wide variations as a consequence of local priorities or incompetent local managers. In time we may come to expect inequalities in healthcare as we do inequalities in the services provided by local government.

At some point these issues will need to be faced. It seems likely that the role that government will want citizens to play in future will be to legitimise decisions about priorities and which services should be provided by the NHS. If the future role of the NHS and local government is commissioning public services, it is likely that they will explicitly want participation in making these choices. This requires an understanding of the purpose of healthcare for individuals and society (Hill, 1996). It requires an open dialogue between citizens and the state with participation and transparency in information, accountability and decision-making. The question remains about mechanisms needed to share healthcare resources equitably across populations and how the public, as citizens and as service users, can be involved in these decisions.

Arrangements for participation, such as LINks, may ensure that a wide range of voices are heard in determining decisions on priorities and in that way decisions are more likely to be seen as 'fair' by local communities. Participation may also be used to educate citizens on the need to balance the idea of individual rights to services with their responsibilities in terms of compliance. However, it is possible that the needs of socially stigmatised groups, such as substance users, overweight people, migrants and undocumented people, may no longer be met. Cuts that affect the most vulnerable may be implemented in the name of local community preferences and voters demands. This is especially likely in the absence of a robust public health function with the capacity to carry out and publicise population needs assessment.

It remains to be seen how willing citizens will be to engage in these decisions. But the debate needs to be public, explicit and transparent. It will not be enough to rely on those who are organised and articulate and those who can speak loudly. While it seems likely that assistance in rationing decisions will be what the NHS will want from LINks, they may not deliver this, particularly if the government and the NHS are not willing to explicitly acknowledge that this is what they want. Credible arrangements will be needed to ensure that people whose views are not normally heard can take part. There will also be the need to develop and maintain a strong presence for user and public interest voices at national level, which governments view with ambivalence, as evidenced by the fate of ACHCEW and the Association of Health Councils in Scotland.

Tackling inequalities and social rights

The consumerist agenda may lead to an increase in inequalities and injustices within society. Decisions about eligibility for treatment may also lead to decisions that will most adversely effect people at the margins of society or who are already vulnerable and disadvantaged. The danger of empowering communities is that the voices that are heard may be used to justify discrimination against some groups, or for not providing services for some people. This is a long way from the original ideals of the NHS.

Perhaps the biggest challenge is how to make sure that arrangements for participation do not reinforce inequalities. If all parts of the community are to have opportunities to be involved, there will need to be outreach, support and training. It is much easier and cheaper to rely on existing users and the

---

Box 11.1   Three key features of human rights

1. They belong to everyone – because we are all human. Human rights focus on what unites us, rather than what divides us.
2. They are principally about the relationships between people and the state. They are not only about protecting us from the abuses of state power, but are also about the state having positive duties to promote and help fulfil people's rights. But human rights can also help to create binding ties between people through the notion that everyone has a responsibility to respect each other's rights.
3. They are a 'floor', but are not a 'ceiling': they are the entitlements that we should all have to flourish as human beings.

Source: Ghose and Weir, 2007.

'usual suspects'. Participation needs to be linked with equity within a framework of social rights. Social rights have been eclipsed by consumer rights. Human rights legislation has largely been used in health and social care to argue for consumer rights, but could be a framework to tackle discrimination and poverty and reinvigorate democracy – especially among people in society whose voices are rarely heard – but only if the legislation were expanded to include social and economic rights (see Box 11.1) (Ghose and Weir, 2007).

A fundamental error that can be made is to believe that user involvement can be managed and voices captured. It can be facilitated but trends towards managing participation will ultimately fail because people become cynical. Participation has to be for some purpose and too often it seems to be a management tool to be disposed of when it does not produce the goods.

In England local involvement networks have to overcome scepticism following eight years of disruption, false dawns and dashed hopes. There are possibilities once again for a new start in England by linking patient and public involvement with citizen engagement, and local involvement networks provide the possibility of doing this. However, this can only happen if participation is linked with equity and social rights and not seen as a process to be managed.

Notes

Chapter 2   The Story Begins

1   Quoted in Smith, D. Aneurin Bevan and the World of South Wales. Cardiff: University of Wales Press, 1973.
2   CHC News, No 42, May, 1979: 11.

Chapter 3   Community Health Councils – The Rise 1974–1979

1   Tory Views on CHCs. CHC News, No 25, 1977.
2   LJ Bowling, CHCs and Realism. CHC News, No. 42, May 1979: 5.

Chapter 4   Community Health Councils – The Decline 1979–1997

1   Tory Views on CHCs. CHC News, No 25, 1977.
2   Helen Hunter, 'Running with the hares'. *Health Service Journal*, 11 July 1996: 11.
3   Barbara Millar, 'On goes the Muzzle', *Health Service Journal*, 28 November 1996: 11.
4   Attempts were made to obtain a copy of this report, but it was not possible to trace it through the Scottish Office, or other national bodies. This information was provided by several informants.

Chapter 5   Tackling the Democratic Deficit

1   Jeanette Mitchell, 'Consultation or…Community action?' *CHC News*, No. 44, July 1979.
2   Jo Revill, 'Sham' Citizens juries face controls. The Observer, 30 September 2007: 23.

Chapter 6   The Rise of Consumer Rights

1   CHC News, CHCs at Work. December 1977: 6–7.
2   Figures obtained by the BBC under the Freedom of Information Act in 2006 showed that 55 percent of complaints had been with the Healthcare Commission or more than six months and of those, nearly 900 complaints had spent more than a year at this second stage of review. BBC Report, Monday, 4 September 2006, accessed www.bbc.co.uk 15 March 2007.
3   'Professional Regulation: Doctors Who Don't Deliver', *Health Service Journal*, 17 April 1997: 24–6
4   Baby Charlotte faces foster care as parents can't cope, Daily Mail, 16th October 2006.
5   Sarah Kate Templeton, Charities get 'covert' aid from drug firms. Sunday Times, 3 December 2006.
6   Nick Stace, This Drugs TV Could Wreak Havoc on Our Health Services. The Guardian, 29 May 2007.

Chapter 7   Promoting Health

1   Health Matters, Issue 37, Summer 1999, page 3.
2   CHC News, No. 74, March 1982.
3   Department of Health. Helping Patients to Take Control of Long Term Illnesses. Press Release, 2 April 2007.
4   Community Health News, 3 January 1985.

Chapter 8   Past Imperfect...Abolishing CHCs

1   CHCs Face a Shake-up After Damning Report. *Health Service Journal*, 2 July 1998: 7.
2   Pat Healy, Role call. *Health Service Journal*, 23 July 1998: 12–13.
3   Patrick Butler, Pastures new. *Health Service Journal*, 11 June 1998: 11–12.
4   Pat Healy, Role call. *Health Service Journal*, 23 July 1998: 12–13.
5   Pat Healy, CHCs join revolt over director appointment. *Health Service Journal*, 18 June 1998: 4.
6   Staff and Patients to Shape the Future of the NHS. Press Release 12 April 2000. London: Department of Health.
7   Reports from this working group were not available from the Department of Health under Freedom of Information and members had been asked to destroy all the papers they received as they were considered to be sensitive. This information came from the recollection of members and civil servants.
8   Peter Walsh. Another Brick in the Wall. *Health Service Journal*, 1 November 2001: 26–7.
9   L Greenwood, Barking Mad. *Health Service Journal*, 13 July 2000: 18.
10 South Birmingham CHC (2003) Trumpet Voluntary: An Informal History of Central and South Birmingham Community Health Councils in 1974 to 2003. South Birmingham CHC.
11 Letter from Alan Milburn, Secretary of State for Health to Donna Covey, ACHCEW Director, 5 October 2000, obtained under the Freedom of Information Act.
12 Parliamentary Question No 136897, 15 November 2000.
13 Michael White, It's a Dog's Life as CHCs Refuse to Lie Down and Die. *Health Service Journal*, 30 November 2001: 21.
14 Tony Tester, End the State of Limbo CHC Have Been in Since the NHS Plan was published, letter, *Health Service Journal*, 8 March 2002: 22–3.
15 David Batty Patients' Watchdog Overhaul. Society Guardian, 3 September, 2001, www.SocietyGuardian.co.uk
16 Evolution Not Abolition for CHCs. *Health Service Journal*, 16 August 2001: 5.
17 House of Lords, Hansard 11 Apr 2002: Column 585, Column 579.
18 Patient and Public Involvement Transition Advisory Board, Objectives and Terms of Reference. Department of Health, undated.
19 Department of Health, Response to the Interim report of the Transition Advisory Board, letter from Rob Thompson, Head of Patient and Public Involvement, Department of Health to Paul Streets, Chair of the Transition Advisory Board, 2 October 2002.
20 Minutes of the tenth and final meeting of the Transition Advisory Board held on 4th December 2002 at Richmond House, Department of Health, London, attached paper. The lessons of the Transitional Advisory Board (TAB) for the Department of Health's involvement of stakeholders. London, Transition Advisory Board.
21 Letter from Sarah Mullally, Chief Nursing Officer, to Strategic Health Authorities, 12 September 2002.

Chapter 9   The Second Coming – The Commission and Patients' Forums

1   Ian Brittain, Barrie Taylor, Suzanne Tyler. Contributory Factors. *Health Service Journal*, 2 May 2002: 30–1.
2   Camden CHC. *Involving the Community in Health: Learning the Lessons in Camden*, November 2003.

3   Nick Edwards, Abolition? It's Nothing Personal. *Health Service Journal*, 4 February 2005: 18–19.
4   Commission for Patient and Public Involvement in Health, Minutes of a Board Meeting held on 29th May 2003.
5   In-fighting Hits CHC Handover. *Health Service Journal*, 10 July 2003: 9.
6   Stephen O'Brien MP, 23 Jun 2003: Hansard, Column 833.
7   Motion to Resolve (Earl Howe), Withdrawn, [644] (13.2.03) 884–902. Commission for Patient and Public Involvement in Health (Functions) Regulations 2002.
8   Motion to Resolve (Earl Howe), Withdrawn, [644] (13.2.03) 884–902. Commission for Patient and Public Involvement in Health (Functions) Regulations 2002.
9   Hugh Muir. Preparation for Patients Forums in Crisis. *The Guardian*, 27 October 2003.
10 *Health Service Journal*, Forums Lose Support as Contracts are Cut. 21 April 2004: 8.
11 David Brindle, Stood up, Stood Down. *Society Guardian*, 23 March 2005: 6–7.
12 Geoff Watts, Second Coming for Patient Power. *British Medical Journal*, 326, 8 March 2003.
13 Commission for Patient and Public Involvement in Health 2003–04 Annual Report. Ordered by the House of Commons to be printed 23 May 2005.
14 Commission for Patient and Public Involvement in Health 2003–04 Annual Report. Ordered by the House of Commons to be printed 20 July 2005.
15 Patients Forums' Battle for Cash and Back-up. *Health Service Journal*, 8 April 2004.
16 Patients Forums' Battle for Cash and Back-up'. *Health Service Journal*, 8 April 2004.
17 Anger Over High Pay at CPPIH. *Health Service Journal*, 7 December 2006: 12.
18 Anger Over High Pay at CPPIH. *Health Service Journal*, 7 December 2006: 12.
19 Evidence submitted by Mike Cox to the Health Committee on Patient and Public Involvement in the NHS. 2007, Volume II: 227.
20 Janet Albu, Regarding Complaints: A Report to the Network of London Forums, 12 September 2006.
21 H Gaze. Forums Lose 11 percent of their Members. *Health Service Journal*, 17 June 2004: 8–9.
22 Nick Edwards, Abolition? It's Nothing Personal. *Health Service Journal*, 24 February 2005:18–19.
23 Commission for Patient and Public Involvement in Health, Board Minutes of the meeting held on 25 March 2004.
24 Evidence submitted by the Shaw Trust to the Health Committee on Patient and Public Involvement in the NHS. 2007, Volume II: 294.
25 YFA Consultancy and Training (2005) Making a *Difference – Diversity Audit for CPPIH*. London YFA Consultancy and Training. Unpublished, obtained under the Freedom of Information Act.
26 Commission for Patient and Public Involvement in Health, Annual Report and Accounts 2005–06.
27 Unease at Forums' Influence, *Health Service Journal*, 17 February 2005: 8.
28 Hampstead and Highgate Express. *Volunteers Quit Health Watchdog Following 'Threat'*. Hampstead and Highgate Express. 25 March 2005: 28.
29 Hampstead and Highgate Express. *Volunteers Quit Health Watchdog Following 'Threat'*. Hampstead and Highgate Express. 25 March 2005: 28.
30 Malcolm Alexander, *Unhealthy Bodies*. Letter Private Eye 11–24 June 2004, Vol. 1108.
31 Private Eye, News 1- 14 October 2004, Vol. 1101.
32 Christine Hogg, *Patient and Public Involvement in Health –What Happens Next? Implications of the Abolition of the CPPIH. Discussion Paper Based on Feedback from National Organisations*. Commissioned by the Department of Health and CPPIH, 2004, unpublished.
33 Commission for Patient and Public Involvement in Health, Minutes of a Board Meeting held on 29 May 2003.
34 Commission for Patient and Public Involvement in Health 2004–05 Annual Report. Ordered by the House of Commons to be printed 20 July 2005.
35 Commission for Patient and Public Involvement in Health 2005–06 Annual Report. Ordered by the House of Commons to be printed 20 July 2005.

36 Hansard 15 Nov 2004: Column 1161W.

37 Hansard 29 Oct 2003: Column 241W.

38 Professor Celia Davies, Evidence to the Health Select Committee, 2007, Volume 1: 31.

39 Commission for Patient and Public Involvement in Health 2003–04 Annual Report. Ordered by the House of Commons to be printed 20 July 2005.

Chapter 10 Renewing Democracy

1 Ian McCartney, *Keep Your Nerve: This is the Rebuilding of Popular Socialism*. The Guardian, 2 December 2002.

2 *Criticism for Public Consultation Bill. Health Service Journal*, 6 January 2007: 6.

3 *Public Consultation Costs Could Hit £1.24m, Health Services Journal*, 24 November 2005: 6.

4 Joe Farrington-Douglas, Signs *of the Times: Will People Power Deliver Accountability? Health Service Journal*, 27 July 2006: 14–15.

5 Report of the Conservative Party Summit on Patient and Public Engagement; Thursday 26th October 2006.

6 Anna Coote, Healthcare Commission, Evidence to the House of Commons Select Committee on PPI, 2007: 39.

7 Elizabeth Manero, Healthlink, Evidence to the House of Commons Select Committee on PPI, 2007: 38.

8 Department of Health Press release, LINks bill given Royal assent, 31 October 2007.

9 Lords sever LINks with NHS. *Health Service Journal*, 25 October 2007: 15.

10 House of Commons Health Select Committee on Patient and Public Involvement, 2007: 69.

11 Evidence to the House of Commons Select Committee on PPI, 2007: 55–7.

12 Letter from Michael McGimpsey, Minister of Health, Social Services and Public Safety, Review of Public Administration, Health and Social Care. February 2008. Belfast: Department of Health, Social Services and Public Safety.

13 Cliff Prior, There may be answers, but what is the question? New Statesman Supplement Healthcare and the Third Sector, 16 July 2007: 4–5.

14 Peter Cardy, *Across the Great Divide*, 8 November 2006, Guardian Society, Charities: 1–2.

Chapter 11 Conclusions

1 Sally Gainsbury, Nicholson signals patients to get hold of purse strings. *Health Service Journal*, 22 November 2007: 9.

Further Reading

Health policy

Baggott, R. (2007) *Understanding Health Policy*. Bristol: the Policy Press.

Ham, C. (2004) Health Policy in Britain: The Politics and Organisation of the National Health Service (Public Policy and Politics). Basingstoke: Macmillan.

Hogg, C. (1999) *Patients, Power and Politics*. London: Sage.

Jones, K. (2000) *The Making of Social Policy in Britain*. London: The Athlone Press.

Klein, R. (2001) *The New Politics of the NHS*. 4th Edition. Harlow: Prentice Hall.

Participation

Beresford, P. (2002) 'Participation and Social Policy: Transformation, Liberation or Regulation?' that in R. Sykes, C. Bochel, and N. Ellison, *Social Policy Review*, 14: 265–87.

Crawford, M., Rutter, D., Thelwell, S. (2003) *User Involvement in Change Management: A Review of the Literature*. Report to the National Co-ordinating Centre for NHS Service Delivery and Organisation R&D. London: NCCSDO. http://www.sdo.lshtm.ac.uk/

Farrell, C. (2004) *Patient and Public Involvement in Health: the Evidence the Policy Implementation, a Summary of the Results of the Health in Partnership Research Programme*. London: Department of Health.

Hogg, C. (1999) *Patients, Power and Politics*. London: Sage.

Lowndes, V., Pratchett, L. and Stoker, G. (2001a) 'Trends in Public Participation, Part 1: Local Government Perspectives'. *Public Administration*, 79 (1): 205–22.

Lowndes, V., Pratchett, L. and Stoker, G. (2001b) 'Trends in Public Participation, Part 2: Citizens' Perspectives'. *Public Administration*, 79 (2): 445–55.

Lupton, C., Peckham, S. and Taylor, P. (1998) *Managing Public Involvement in Healthcare Purchasing*. Buckingham: Open University Press.

Rose, D., Fleishmann, P., Tonkiss, F., Campbell, P. and Wykes, T. (2002) *User Involvement in Change Management in a Mental Health Context – A Review of the Literature*. London: National Co-ordinating Centre for NHS Service Delivery and Organisational R&D (NCCSDO). http://www.sdo.lshtm.ac.uk/

Complaints and individual choices

Allsop, J. and Mulcahy, L. (1996) Regulating Medical Work: Formal and Informal Controls. Buckingham: Open University Press.

Needham, C. (2003) *Citizen-consumers – New Labour's Marketplace Democracy. London: Catalyst* www.catalstforum.org.uk

Promoting health

Baggott, R. (2000) *Public Health: Policy and Politics*. Basingstoke: Palgrave.

Hunter, D.J. (2004) *Public Health Policy*. Cambridge: Polity.

Ghose, K. and Weir, S. (2007) *Human Rights, A Tool for Change*. London: ESRC.

Naidoo, J. and Wills, J. (2004) Health and Health Promotion: developing practice. London : Bailliere Tindall ; RCN.

Community health councils

Gerrard, M. (2006) *A Stifled Voice*. Brighton: Pen Press.

Klein, R. and Lewis, J. (1976) *The Politics of Consumer Representation: A Study of Community Health Councils*. London: Centre for Studies in Social Policy.

CHC News 1975–1983. Available at the King's Fund Library. The Welcome Library and Oxford Brookes University also hold archives.

Voluntary sector

Baggott, R., Allsop, J. and Jones, K. (2005) *Speaking for Patients and Carers: Health Consumer Groups and the Policy Process*. Basingstoke: Palgrave Macmillan.

References

ACHCEW (1989) *Effective CHCs in the 1990s: Report of a Panel of Inquiry.* London: Association of CHCs for England and Wales.

ACHCEW (1993) *Rationing Health Care: Should Community Health Councils Help?* London: Association of CHCs for England and Wales.

ACHCEW (1997) *A Stronger Voice for Patients in the New Millennium: Response to the INSIGHT Report.* London: Association of CHCs for England and Wales.

ACHCEW (2003) *A Friend in Need.* London: Association of CHCs for England and Wales.

Acheson, D. (1998) *Inequalities in Health: Report of an Independent Inquiry.* London: Stationery Office.

Agass, M., Coulter, A., Mant, D. and Fuller, A. (1991) 'Patient Participation in General Practice: Who Participates?' *British Journal of General Practice,* 41: 198–201.

Alford, J. (1998) A Public Management Road Less Travelled: Clients and Co-producers of Public Services. *Australian Journal of Public Administration,* 57 (4): 128–37.

Anderson, W. and Florin, D. (2000) *Involving the Public – One of Many Priorities: A Survey of Public Involvement in London's Primary Care Groups.* King's Fund London.

Arnold, C., Etherington, P. and Taylor, B. (1995a) *CHCs at the Millennium: the Views of CHC Members.* No publisher. Accessed at the Oxford Brookes University ACHCEW Archives'.

Arnold, C., Etherington, P. and Taylor, B. (1995b) *CHCs at the Millennium: A Strategic Discussion Paper.* Burnley, Pendale and Rossendale CHC.

Arnold, C., Finucane, A., Lee, N. and Taylor, B. (1992) *Self Review in CHCs: Facilitator's Manual.* London: ACHCEW.

Arnstein, S.R. (1969) 'A ladder of citizen participation'. *Journal of the American Institute of Planners,* 35: 216–24 July.

Baggott, R. (2005) 'A Funny Thing Happened on the Way to the Forum? Reforming Patient and Public Involvement in the NHS in England'. *Public Administration,* 83 (3): 2005.

Baggott, R. (2007) Understanding Health Policy. Bristol: the Policy Press.

Baggott, R., Allsop, J. and Jones, K. (2005) *Speaking for Patients and Carers: Health Consumer Groups and the Policy Process.* Basingstoke: Palgrave Macmillan.

Barker, I., Newbiggin, K. and Peck, E. (1997) 'Characteristics for Sustained Advocacy Projects in Mental Health Services'. *Community Care Management and Planning Review,* 5 (4): 132–9.

Barnes, M. (1999) 'Users and Citizens: Collective Action and the Local Governance of Welfare'. *Social Policy and Administration,* 33 (1): 73–90.

Barnes, M. (2002) 'Bringing a Difference into Deliberation? Disabled People, Survivors and Local Government'. *Policy and Politics,* 30(3): 319–31.

Barrett, A., Roques, T., Small, M. and Smith, R.D. (2006) 'How Much Will Herceptin Really Cost?' *British Medical Journal,* 333: 1118–20.

Bate, R. and Robert, G. (2005) 'Choice: More Can Mean Less', *British Medical Journal,* 331: 1488–9.

Bates, E. (1982) 'Can the Public's Voice Influence Bureaucracy? The Case of Community Health Councils.' *Public Administration,* 60 (1): 92–8.

Beresford, P. (2002) 'Participation and Social Policy: Transformation, Liberation or Regulation?' in R. Sykes, C. Bochel, and N. Ellison, *Social Policy Review,* 14: 265–87.

Blackmore, A. (2004) *Standing Apart, Working Together: A Study of the Myths and Realities of Voluntary and Community Sector Independence.* London: NCVO.

Blackmore, A. (2006) *The Reform of Public Services: The Role of the Voluntary Sector.* London: National Council for Voluntary Organisations.

BMA (2007) *A Rational Way Forward for the NHS in England: A Discussion Paper Outlining an Alternative Approach to Health Reform.* London: British Medical Association.

BME Health Forum (2006) *Minding the Gaps: Are BME Groups Partners or Substitutes in Health Provision? Research into the Participation of BME Organisations and Groups in Health*

Consultations and Activities in Kensington, Chelsea and Westminster. London: BME Health Forum.

Bolzan, N. and Gale, F. (2002) 'The Citizenship of Excluded Groups: Challenging the Consumerist Agenda'. *Social Policy and Administration* 36 (4): 363–75.

Boyd, J. (2007) The 2006 Inpatients Importance Study. Oxford: Picker Institute Europe.

Bridge Consultancy (1998) *In the Public Interest: Developing a Strategy for Public Participation in the NHS.* Cambridge: The Bridge Consultancy.

Brown, P. and Zavestoski, S. (2004) 'Social Movements in Health: An Introduction'. *Sociology of Health and Illness,* 26(6): 679–94.

Buckland, S., Lupton, C. and Moon, G. (1995) *An Evaluation of the Role and Impact of Community Health Councils.* Social Services Research and Information Unit. Portsmouth: Portsmouth University.

Calnan, M. and Gabe, J. (2001) 'From Consumerism to Partnership? Britain's National Health Service at the Turn of the Century'. *International Journal of Health Services,* 31 (1): 119–31.

Campbell, F. (2005) *Health Scrutiny Works! A Review of Effective Local Authority Scrutiny of Health in its First Two Years.* London: Democratic Health Network.

Campbell, P. (1996) 'The History of the User Movement in the UK'. In T. Heller et al. (eds) *Mental Health Matters,* 218–25, Basingstoke: Macmillan.

Carrington, D. (2005) 'Financing the Voluntary and Community Sector – Future Prospects and Possibilities'. In *Voluntary Action: Meeting the Challenges of the 21st Century,* pp. 95–117. London: National Council for Voluntary Organisations.

Chandler, D. (2001) 'Active Citizens and the Therapeutic State: the Role of Democratic Participation in Local Government Reform'. *Policy and Politics* 29 (1): 2–14.

CHI (2004) *i2i Involvement to Improvement: Sharing the Learning about Patient and Public Involvement from CHI's Inspections.* London: Commission for Health Improvement.

Chisholm, A., Redding, D., Cross, P. and Coulter, A. (2007) *Patient and Public Involvement in PCT Commissioning: A Survey of Primary Care Trusts.* Oxford: Picker Institute.

Citizens Advice (2005) *The Pain of Complaining: CAB ICAS Evidence of the NHS Complaints Procedure.* London: Citizens Advice.

Consumers International (2006) *Branding the Cure: A Consumer Perspective on Corporate Social Responsibility, Drug Promotion and the Pharmaceutical Industry in Europe.* London: Consumers International.

Cooke, B. and Kothari, U. (2001) *Participation: the New Tyranny?* London: Zed.

Cooper, L., Coote, A., Davies, A., Jackson, C. (1996) *Voices Off? Tackling the Democratic Deficit in Health.* London: Institute for Public Policy Research

Coote, A. and Lenaghan, J. (1997) Citizens' juries: Theory into Practice, London: Institute of Public Policy Research.

Coulter, A. (2002) *The Autonomous Patient: Ending Paternalism in Medical Care.* London: Nuffield Trust.

Coulter, A. (2006) *Engaging Patients in their Healthcare: How is the UK Doing Relative to Other Countries?* Oxford: Picker Institute.

Craig, G., Taylor, M., and Parkes, T. (2004) 'Protest or Partnership? The Voluntary and Community Sectors in the Policy Process'. *Social Policy and Administration,* 38 (30): 221–39.

Crawford, M., Rutter, D., Manley, C., Weaver, T., Bhui, K., Falop, N. and Tyrer, P. (2002) 'Systematic Review of Involving Patients in the Planning and Development of Health Care'. *British Medical Journal,* 325: 1263–7.

Crinson, I. (1998) Putting Patients First: the Continuity of the Consumerist Discourse in Health Policy, From Radical Right to New Labour. *Critical Social Policy,* 18 (2): 227–39.

Crow, A. (2002) 'Councillors' Attitudes Towards Participation – Kidderminster General Hospital – A Case Study'. *Local Governance,* 28 (2): 115–24.

CSV (2004) *Giving Time: Impact on Health.* London: Community Service Volunteers.

Curtis, H. and Sanderson, M. (2004) *The Unsung Sixties: Memoirs of Social Innovation.* London: Whiting and Birch.

Dabbs, C. (1998) *At the Crossroads – the Future of Community Health Councils.* London: School for Social Entrepreneurs.

Dahlgren, G. and Whitehead, M. (1991) *Policies and Strategies to Promote Social Equity in Health*. Stockholm: Institute of Future Studies.

Davies C., Wetherell, M., Barnett, E. and Seymour-Smith, S. (2005) *Opening the Box: Evaluating the Citizens Council of NICE*. Report prepared for the National Co-ordinating Centre for Research Methodology, NHS R&D Programme (www.pcpoh.bham.ac.uk/publichealth/nccrm/publications.htm).

Davies, C., Wetherell, M. and Barnett, E. (2006) *Citizens at the Centre: Deliberative Participation in Healthcare Decisions*. Bristol: The Policy Press.

Day, P. and Klein, R. (2005) *Governance of Foundation Trusts: Dilemmas of Diversity*. London: The Nuffield Trust.

Day, P. and Klein, R. (2007) *The Politics of Scrutiny: Reconfiguration in NHS England*. London: The Nuffield Trust.

DCLG (2006) *Strong and Prosperous Communities, White Paper*. London: Department of Communities and Local Government.

Deakin, N. (2005) 'Civil Society and Civil Renewal' In *Voluntary Action: Meeting the Challenges of the 21st Century*. pp. 13–46. London: NCVO.

DH (1989) *Working for Patients*. London: Department of Health.

DH (1992) *The Health of the Nation: A Strategy for Health in England*. London: HMSO.

DH (1994a) The Operation of CHCs. EL. (94) 4. London: Department of Health.

DH (1994b) *Being Heard: The Report of a Review Committee on NHS Complaints Procedures*. London: HMSO.

DH (1995) *Community Health Councils: Guidance on the Changes in the Establishing Arrangements*. EL (95) 142. London: Department of Health.

DH (1997) *The New NHS – Modern and Dependable*. London: HMSO.

DH (1998a) *The Health of the Nation – A Policy Assessed*. Two reports commissioned by the Department of Health from the Universities of Leeds and Glamorgan and the London School of Tropical Health and Medicine. London: Stationery Office.

DH (1998b) *Healthy Living Centres*: Report of a conference held on 2 April 1998. London: Stationery Office.

DH (1999) *Saving Lives: Our Healthier Nation*. London: Department of Health

DH (2000) *The NHS Plan: A Plan for Investment, A Plan for Reform*. London: Stationery Office.

DH (2001a) *The Expert Patient: A New Approach to Chronic Disease Management for the 21st century*. London: Department of Health.

DH (2001b) *Shifting the Balance of Power*. London: Department of Health.

DH (2001c) *Involving Patients and the Public in Healthcare: a Discussion Document*. London: Department of Health.

DH (2001d) *Involving Patients and the Public in Healthcare: Response to the Listening Exercise*. London: Department of Health.

DH (2003a) *Improving Chronic Disease Management*. London: Department of Health.

DH (2003b) *Strengthening Accountability. Involving Patients and the Public – Policy and Practice Guidance. Section 11 of the Health and Social Care Act 2001*. London: Department of Health.

DH (2004a) *Choosing Health: Making Healthy Choices Easier*. London: Department of Health.

DH (2004b) *Reconfiguring the Department of Health's Arms Length Bodies*. London: Department of Health.

DH (2006) *On the State of the Public Health: Annual Report of the Chief Medical Officer 2005*. London: Department of Health.

DH (2006a) *Our Health, Our Care, Our Say: A New Direction for Community Services*. London: Department of Health.

DH (2006b) *Concluding the Review of Patient and Public Involvement – Recommendations to Ministers from the Expert Panel*. London Department of Health.

DH (2006c) *A Stronger Local Voice: A Framework for Creating a Stronger Local Voice in the Development of Health and Social Care Services*. London: Department of Health.

DH (2006d) *Commissioning Framework for the English NHS*. London: Department of Health.

DH (2006e) *Reward and Recognition: The Principles and Practice of Service User Payment and Reimbursement in Health and Social Care*. London: Department of Health.

DH (2007a) Making Experiences Count: A New Approach to Responding to Complaints. London: Department of Health.

DH (2007b) Getting Ready for LINks: Contracting a Host Organisation for your Local Involvement Network. London: Department of Health.

DHSS (1970) *The National Health Service: the Future Structure of the NHS.* London: HMSO.

DHSS (1971) *NHS Reorganisation: Consultative Document.* London: Department of Health and Social Security.

DHSS (1974a) *Democracy in the NHS: Membership of Health Authorities.* London: Department of Health and Social Security.

DHSS (1974b) *NHS Reorganisation Circular,* HRC (74)4.

DHSS (1975) *Report of the National Advisers on CHCs.* In Gerrard, 2006.

DHSS (1976a) *Priorities for Health and Personal Social Services in England: A Consultative Document.* London: HMSO.

DHSS (1976b) *Fit for the Future* (Court Report). London: HMSO.

DHSS (1976c) *Prevention and Health: Everybody's Business: A Reassessment of Public and Personal Health.* London: HMSO.

DHSS (1979) *Patient First.* London: HMSO.

DHSS (1980) *Patients First: Summary of Comments Received on the Consultative Paper.* London: Department of Health and Social Security.

DHSS (1981) *The Role of Community Health Councils.* London: Department of Health and Social Security.

DHSS (1983) *NHS Management Inquiry* (Griffiths Report). London: Department of Health and Social Security.

DHSS (1984) Voluntary Organisation Representatives on Joint Consultative Committees and the Extension of Joint Finance Arrangements. HC (84) 9. London: Department of Health and Social Security.

DHSS (1985) *Statutory Instruments the Community Health Council Regulations,* March. London. Department of Health and Social Security.

DHSSPS (2007) *Health and Social Services (Reform) (Northern Ireland) Order. Statutory Instrument.* Belfast: Department of Health, Social Services and Public Safety.

Dixon, M. (1989) 'The Case for a Counter Bureaucracy'. In *Community/Consumer Representation in the NHS with Specific Reference to CHCs,* C. Hogg and F. Winkler (eds). London: the Greater London Association of Community Health Councils.

Doyal, L. with Pennell, I. (1979) The Political Economy of Health. London: Pluto Press.

Duckenfield, M. and Rangnekar, D. (2004) *The Rise of Patients' groups and Drug Development: Towards a Science of Patient Involvement.* London: School of Public Policy University College London.

Dunford, A. (1977) Planning for the consumer: the views of CHCs. Dissertation for MA in social service planning, Colchester, Essex University.

Dyke, G. (1998) *A New NHS Charter – a Different Approach: Report on the New NHS Charter.* London: Department of Health.

Elliott, E., Williams, G.H., and Rolfe, B. (2004) 'The Role of Lay Knowledge in Health Impact Assessment'. In *Health Impact Assessment* J. Kemm and S. Palmer (eds), Oxford: Oxford University Press.

Farrell, C. (2004) *Patient and Public Involvement in Health: the Evidence the Policy Implementation, a Summary of the Results of the Health in Partnership Research Programme.* London: Department of Health.

Farrell, C. and Adams, J. (1981) *CHCs at Work 1980.* London: Department of Applied Social Studies, Polytechnic of North London.

Farrell, C., Levenson, R. and Snape, D. (1998) *The Patients Charter: Past and Present.* London: King's Fund.

Farrington-Douglas, J. and Allen. J. (2005) *Equitable Choices for Health.* London: IPPR.

Faulks, K. (1998) *Citizenship in Modern Britain.* Edinburgh: Edinburgh University Press.

Fishkin, J.S. (1991) *Democracy and Deliberation: New Directions for Democratic Reform.* Yale University Press.

FMR Research (2008) Patient Partnership Forums: What Direction and Support is needed for the Future? A Report Commissioned by the Scottish Health Council. Glasgow: FMR Research.

Foresight (2007) *Tackling Obesities: Future Choice*. London: Department of Innovation, Universities and Skills.

Gerrard, M. (2006) *A Stifled Voice*: *Community Health Councils in England 1974–2003*. Brighton: Pen Press.

Ghose, K. and Weir, S. (2007) *Human Rights, A Tool for Change*. London: ESRC.

Gilchrist, A. (2007) 'Community Development and Networking for Health'. In *Public Health for the 21st Century: New Perspectives on Policy, Participation and Practice*. J. Orme, J. Powell, P. Taylor, and M. Grey (eds). 2nd edition. Maidenhead: McGraw Hill, pp. 135–52.

Greer, S.L. (2004a) *Four Way Bet: How Devolution Has Led to Four Different Models of the NHS*. London, the Constitution Unit, School of Public Policy, University College London.

Greer, S.L. (2004b) *Territorial Politics and Health Policy*. Manchester: Manchester University Press.

Greer, S.L. and Jarman, H. (2007) *The Department of Health and the Civil Service*. London: the Nuffield Trust.

Griffiths, C., Foster, G., Ramsey, J., Elridge, S. and Taylor, S. (2007) 'How Effective are Expert Patient (Lay Led) Education Programmes for Chronic Disease', *British Medical Journal*, 334: 1254–6, 16 June.

Hallas, J. (1976) *CHCs in Action*. London: Nuffield Provincial Hospitals Trust.

Halvorsen, R. (2007) *The Truth About Vaccines: How We are Used as Guinea Pigs without knowing it*. London: Gibson Square.

Harris, T. (1995) 'Securing CHC Independence'. In *CHCs at the Millennium: A Strategic Discussion Paper*. C. Arnold, P. Etherington and B. Taylor. Burnley, Pendale and Rossendale CHC.

Harrison, S. and Mort, M. (1998) 'Which Champions, Which People? Public and User Involvement in Health Care as a Technology of Legitimation?' *Social Policy and Administration*, 32 (1): 60–70.

Healthcare Commission (2005) *The Healthcare Commission's Review of NHS Foundation Trusts*. London: Healthcare Commission.

Hill, T.P. (1996) 'Healthcare: A Social Contract in Transition'. *Social Science and Medicine*. 41 (5): 783–9.

HM Treasury and the Cabinet Office (2006) The Future of the Third Sector in Social and Economic Regeneration. London: HM Treasury and the Cabinet Office.

Hodgkin, P. (2005) 'Will Choice Increase Voice?' *Health Matters*, 62: 7.

Hogg, C. (1986) *The Public and the NHS*. London: Association of CHCs for England and Wales.

Hogg, C. (1987) *Good Practices in CHCs*. London: Association of CHCs for England and Wales.

Hogg, C. (1989) 'A Look Backwards and Forwards'. In *Community/consumer Representation in the NHS with Specific Reference to CHCs*, edited by C. Hogg and F. Winkler. London: the Greater London Association of Community Health Councils.

Hogg, C. (1994a) *Performance Standards for CHCs: Developing the Framework*. London: ACHCEW.

Hogg, C. (1994b) *Beyond the Patients Charter: Working with Users*. London: Health Rights.

Hogg, C. (1995) *Staffing and Resources for Community Health Councils: Report of a Survey*. London: ACHCEW.

Hogg, C. (1996) *Back from the Margins: Which Future for Community Health Councils? Discussion Paper*. London: Institute of Health Services and Management and the Association of Community Health Councils for England and Wales.

Hogg, C. (1999) *Patients, Power and Politics*. London: Sage.

Hogg C. (2004) *Patient and Public Involvement in Health – What Happens Next? Implications of the Abolition of the CPPIH. Discussion Paper Based on Feedback from National Organisations*. Commissioned by the Department of Health and CPPIH, 2004, unpublished.

Hogg, C. (2006a) Interview as part of ESRC research study RES-000-22-1654, 18 October.

Hogg, C. (2006b) Interview with senior civil servant as part of ESRC research study RES-000-22-1654, 19 July.

Hogg, C. (2006c) Interview as part of ESRC research study RES-000-22-1654, 1 November.

Hogg, C. (2006d) Interview as part of ESRC research study RES-000-22-1654, 1 August.

Hogg, C. (2006e) Interview with regional chair as part of ESRC research study RES-000-22-1654, 15 November.

Hogg, C. (2006f) Interview with senior civil servant as part of ESRC research study RES-000-22-1654, 13 October.

Hogg, C. (2006g) Interview of member of ACHCEW management committee as part of ESRC research study RES-000-22-1654, 11 September.

Hogg, C. (2006h) Interview as part of ESRC research study RES-000-22-1654, 23 August.

Hogg, C. (2006i) Interview as part of ESRC research study RES-000-22-1654, 16 August.

Hogg, C. (2006j) Interview with Commissioner as part of ESRC research study RES-000-22-1654, 14 August.

Hogg, C. (2006k) Interview with Commissioner as part of ESRC research study RES-000-22-1654, 6 September.

Hogg, C. (2006l) Interview with regional manager as part of ESRC research study RES-000-22-1654, 13 July.

Hogg, C. (2006m) Interview with regional manager as part of ESRC research study RES-000-22-1654, 29 August.

Hogg, C. (2006n) Interview with Officer at Healthcare Commission as part of ESRC research study RES-000-22-1654, 10 August.

Hogg, C. (2006p) Interview as part of ESRC research study RES-000-22-1654, 30 September.

Hogg, C. (2006q) Interview as part of ESRC research study RES-000-22-1654, 21 October.

Hogg, C. (2007a) Interview as part of ESRC research study RES-000-22-1654, 15 February.

Hogg. C. (2007b) Interview with NHS manager working at national policy level as part of ESRC research study RES-000-22-1654, 28 March.

Hogg, C. (2007c) *Public Involvement at National Level: Options for the Future*. A paper prepared for the Scottish Consumer Council. Edinburgh: Scottish Consumer Council.

Hogg, C. (2007d) 'Patient and Public Involvement: What Next for the NHS?' *Health Expectations*, 10 (2): 129–38.

Hogg, C. (2007e) Interview as part of ESRC research study RES-000-SS-1654, 18 May.

Hogg, C. and Graham, L. (2001) *Patient and Public Involvement in the NHS: What is Needed at National Level*. London: Patients Forum.

Hogg, C. and Joule. N. (1994) *CHCs and Primary Care*. London: Greater London Association of CHCs.

Hogg, C. and Williamson, C. (2001) 'Whose Interests Do Lay People Represent? Towards an Understanding of the Role of Lay People as Members of Committees'. *Health Expectations*, 4(1): 2–9.

Hogg, C., Loosemore-Reppen, G. and Rowan, K. (2006) *The Patients Forum: Options for the Future*. London: The Patients Forum.

Home Office (2005) *Together We Can – Action Plan*. London, Home Office.

House of Commons Health Committee (2001) *Public Health. Second Report. Volume 1 Report and Proceedings of the Committee*. Session 2000–2001. HC30-II. London: Stationery Office.

House of Commons Health Committee (2003) Patient and Public Involvement in the NHS Seventh Report 2002–03. London: the Stationery Office.

House of Commons Health Committee (2007) Patient *and Public Involvement in the NHS*. Third Report 2006–07. Volume I. London: the Stationery Office.

Hunter, D. (1989) 'Introduction'. In *Community/consumer Representation in the NHS with Specific Reference to CHCs*. C. Hogg and F. Winkler (eds). London: the Greater London Association of Community Health Councils.

Hunter, D.J. (2004) *Public Health Policy*. Cambridge: Polity.

Hutton, W. (2000) *New Life for Health: The Commission on the NHS* (chaired by Will Hutton). London: Vintage.

Insight Consulting (1996) *Resourcing and Performance Management In CHCs Final Report*, submitted to the Department of Health. November, No publisher.

Jochum, J., Pratten, B. and Wilding, K. (2005) *Civil Renewal and Active Citizenship – A Guide to the Debate*. London: NCVO.

Jones, K. (2000) *The Making of Social Policy in Britain*. London: The Athlone Press.

JRF (1999) *Social Cohesion and Urban Inclusion for Disadvantaged Neighbourhoods*. York: Joseph Rowntree Trust.

Kelf-Cohen, R. (1973) *British Nationalisation 1945–1973*. London: Macmillan.

Kennedy Report (2001) *Report of the Public Inquiry into Children's Heart Surgery at the Bristol Royal Infirmary 1984–1995*. London: Stationery Office.

King's Fund (1977) *Evidence to the Royal Commission on the National Health Service*. London: King Edward's Hospital Fund for London.

King's Fund (2006) Designing the 'New' NHS: Ideas to Make a Supplier Market Work. Report of an independent working group. London: King's Fund.

Klein, R. (2001) *The New Politics of the NHS*. 4th Edition. Harlow: Prentice Hall.

Klein, R. (2004) 'Too Much of a Good Thing? Over-investing in Public Involvement in the NHS'. *New Economy*, 11 (4): 207–12.

Klein, R. and Lewis, J. (1976) *The Politics of Consumer Representation: A Study of Community Health Councils*. London: Centre for Studies in Social Policy.

Korff, D. (2007) Guaranteeing Liberty or Big Brother: Surveillance in the United Kingdom. London: Human Rights & Social Justice Institute, London Metropolitan University.

Lepine, E. and Sullivan, H. (2007) 'More Local Than Local Government: The Relationship Between Local Government and the Neighbourhood Agenda'. In I. Smith, E. Lepine, M. Taylor, M., *Disadvantaged by Where You Live? Neighbourhood Governance in Contemporary Urban Policy*. Bristol: Policy Press, pp. 83–103.

Levitt, R. (1980) The *People's Voice in the NHS – CHCs after Five Years*. London: King Edward's Hospital Fund for London.

Lewis, J. (1992) 'Providers, Consumers: the State and the Delivery of Health-care Services in the 20th century'. In Wear, A. (ed.) *Medicine in Society: Historical Essays*. Cambridge: Cambridge University Press: 317–45.

Lewis, J. (1995) *The Voluntary Sector, the State and Social Work in Britain: The Charity Organisation Society/Family Welfare Association since 1969*. Aldershot: Edward Elgar.

Lewis, R. (2005a) 'The Sound of Silence', *Public Finance*, May 13–19: 20–3.

Lewis, R. (2005b) *Governing Foundation Trusts: A New Era for Public Accountability*. London: King's Fund www.kingsfund.org.uk

Lewis, R., Hunt, P. and Carson, D. (2006) *Social Enterprise and Community-based Care*. London: King's Fund.

Lodge, G. and Rogers, B. (2006) *Whitehall's Black Box: Accountability and performance in the Senior Civil Service*. London: IPPR.

Lowndes, V., Pratchett, L. and Stoker, G. (2001a) 'Trends in Public Participation, Part 1: Local Government Perspectives'. *Public Administration*, 79(1): 205–22.

Lowndes, V., Pratchett, L. and Stoker, G. (2001b) 'Trends in Public Participation, Part 2: Citizens' Perspectives'. *Public Administration*, 79(2): 445–55.

Lucas, K., Ross, A. and Fuller, S. (2003) What's in a Name? Local Agenda 21, Community Planning and Neighbourhood Renewal. York: Joseph Rowntree Foundation.

Lupton, C., Peckham, S. and Taylor, P. (1998) *Managing Public Involvement in Healthcare Purchasing*. Buckingham: Open University Press.

Lupton, D. (1997) 'Consumerism, Reflexivity and the Medical Encounter'. *Social Science and Medicine*, 45 (3): 373–81.

Lyons Inquiry (2006) *Lyons Inquiry into Local Government: National Prosperity, Local Choice and Civic Engagement: A New Partnership Between Central and Local Government for the 21st century*. London: Stationery Office.

Lyons Inquiry (2007) *Lyons Inquiry into Local Government: Place-shaping: A Shared Ambition for the Future of Local Government*. London: Stationery Office.

Marks, L. and Hunter, D.J. (2007) *Social Enterprises and the NHS: Changing Patterns of Ownership and Accountability*. London: Unison.

Marmot, M. (2004) *Status Syndrome*. London: Bloomsbury.

Marquand, D. (2004) *Decline of the Public: The Hollowing-out of Citizenship*. Cambridge: Polity Press.

Martin, S. et al. (2001) *Improving Local Public Services: Evaluation of the Best Value Pilot Programme, Final report.* London: Department of the Environment, Transport and the Regions.

May, J. (2005) *The Triangle of Engagement: An Unusual Way of Looking at the Usual Suspects.* MPA Community Engagement Unit. Occasional Paper No. 1. London: Metropolitan Police Authority.

McIver, S. (1993) *Investing in Patient's Representatives.* Birmingham: National Association of Health Authorities and Trusts.

Milewa, T., Harrison S. and Dowswell, G. (2003) 'Public Involvement and Democratic Accountability in Primary Care Organisations'. In B. Dowling and C. Glendinning (eds) *The New NHS, Modern, Dependable Successful?* Buckingham: Open University Press.

Mills, F. (2000) *Patients' groups and the Global Pharmaceutical Industry – The Growing Importance of Working Directly with the Consumer.* London: Informa Pharmaceuticals.

Moon, G. and Lupton, C. (1995) 'Within Acceptable Limits: Health Care Provider Perspectives on Community Health Councils in England and Wales', *Policy and Politics*, 23, 4, 335–46.

Muir Gray, J.A. (2001) *Evidence-based Healthcare: How to Make Health Policy and Management Decisions.* London: Churchill Livingstone.

Muir Gray, J.A. (2002) *The Resourceful Patient.* Oxford: eRosetta Press.

NAO (1996a) *Health of the Nation: A Progress Report*, HSC 656 Session 1995–96. London: HMSO.

NAO (1996b) *Improving Health in Wales.* HC 633 1995–1996. London: National Audit Office.

NAPP (2007) *A Survey of Patient Participation Groups in General Practice (2005–2007).* National Association for Patient Participation Groups, www.napp.org.uk

NCC (1997) *NHS Complaints Procedures: the First Year.* London: the National Consumer Council.

NCC (2006) *It's Our Health! Realising the Potential of Effective Social Marketing.* London: National Consumer Council.

NCC and ACHCEW (1984) *Information Needs of CHCs.* London: ACHCEW.

NCVO (1986) *A Stake in Planning: Joint Planning and the Voluntary Sector, Report of the NCVO Joint Planning Working Group.* London, NCVO.

Needham, C. (2003) *Citizen-consumers – New Labour's Marketplace Democracy.* London: Catalyst, www.catalstforum.org.uk

Newman, J., Barnes, M., Sullivan, H. and Knops, A. (2004) 'Public Participation and Collaborative Governance'. *Journal of Social Policy*, 33, 2, 203–23.

NHS Alliance (2007) Practice-based Commissioning and Patient and Public Involvement – The New Frontier. Retford: The NHS Alliance.

NHSE (1996) *Patient Partnership: Building a Collaborative Strategy.* Leeds: NHS Executive.

NHSME (1992) *Local Voices: The Views of Local People in Purchasing for Health.* London: NHS Management Executive.

OLR (2005) *Consultation on the Future Support for Patient and Public Involvement in Health.* Short Report. London: Opinion Leader Research.

Owen, D. (1976) In *Sickness and in Health: the Politics of Medicine.* London: Quartet Books.

Owen, D. (1988) *Our NHS.* London: Pan.

Patients Association (2005) *Patients' Rights in Europe and the UK.* London: the Patients Association.

Peck, E. (1998) 'Integrity, Ambiguity or Duplicity? NHS Consultation with the Public'. *Health Services Management Research*, 11: 201–10.

Peck, E. and Barker, I. (1997) 'Users and Partners in Mental Health – Ten Years of Experience'. *Journal of Interprofessional Care.* 11 (3): 269–77.

Pickard, S. (1998) 'Citizenship and Consumerism in Healthcare: A Critique of Citizens' Juries'. *Social Policy and Administration*, 32 (3): 226–44.

Pickard, S. (1997) 'The Future Organisation of Community Health Councils'. *Social Policy and Administration*, 31 (3) 274–89.

Piette, D. (1985) *A Study of the Contribution of Community Health Councils in Health Education for Children of School Age.* Thesis for M.Phil, London School of Hygiene and Tropical Medicine, June.

Pollock, A. (2004) *NHS Plc: The Privatisation of Our Health Care.* London: Verso.

Power Inquiry (2006) *Power to the People, The Report of Power, An Independent Inquiry into Britain's Democracy.* The centenary project of the Joseph Rowntree Charitable Trust and the Joseph Rowntree Reform Trust. York: the Power Inquiry.

Prior, L. (2003) 'Belief, Knowledge and Expertise: The Emergence of the Lay Expert in Medical Sociology'. *Sociology of Health and Illness,* 25th silver anniversary edition: 41–57.

Pritchard, P. (1994) 'Community Involvement in a Changing World', in Z. Heritage (ed.) *Community Participation in Primary Care.* London: Royal College of General Practitioners.

Richards, N. and Coulter, A. (2007) *Is the NHS Becoming More Patient-centred? Trends from the National Surveys of NHS Patients in England 2002–2007.* Oxford: Picker Institute Europe.

Richardson, A. (1983) *Participation.* London: Routledge and Kegan Paul.

Rolfe, M., Holden, D. and Lawes, H. (1998) *Reflecting the Public Interest: Focused and Professional – A Strategy for CHCs to Plan their Own Future.* No publisher. Accessed at Oxford Brookes University Archive.

Rose, D., Fleishmann, P., Tonkiss, F., Campbell, P. and Wykes, T. (2002) *User Involvement in Change Management in a Mental Health Context – A Review of the Literature.* London: National Co-ordinating Centre for NHS Service Delivery and Organisational R&D (NCCSDO).

Royal Commission on the National Health Service (1979) *Report,* cmnd 7615. London: HMSO.

Sandford, M. (2005) *External Scrutiny: The Voice in the Crowded Room.* London: Centre for Public Scrutiny.

Saunders, D. (1985) *CHC Involvement in District Planning Teams, a Survey of the West Midlands Region in 1984,* unpublished paper, quoted in Hogg (1986).

SCC (2004) *Comments on advice notes on public partnership forums,* Edinburgh: Scottish Consumer Council.

Scottish Executive (2000) *Our National Health: A Plan for Action, A Plan for Change.* Edinburgh: Scottish Executive.

Scottish Executive (2003) *Patient Focus and Patient Involvement.* Edinburgh: Scottish Executive.

Scott-Samuel, A. and Wills, J. (2007) 'Health Promotion in England: Sleeping Beauty or Corpse?' *Health Education Journal,* 66 (2): 115–19.

Sen, A. (2002) 'Health: Perception versus observation'. *British Medical Journal,* 324, 860–1.

Shaw, J. and Baker, M. (2004) 'Expert Patient – Dream or Nightmare?' *British Medical Journal,* 328: 723–4.

Shickle, D. and Chadwick, R. (1994) 'The Ethics of Screening: Is 'Screeningitis' an Incurable Disease?' *Journal of Medical Ethics,* 20: 12–18.

Smee C (2005) *Speaking Truth to Power: Two Decades of Analysis in the Department of Health.* Oxford: Radcliffe Publishing Ltd.

Stoker, G. (2005) 'New Localism and the Future of Local Governance: Implications for the voluntary sector'. *In Voluntary Action: meeting the challenges of the 21st Century,* London NCVO.

TAB (2002a) *Interim Report to the Department of Health,* July. London: Transition Advisory Board.

TAB (2002b) *Public and Patient Involvement in Health: Key Messages for the Commission for Patient and Public Involvement in Health and the Department of Health.* Final Report. December. London: Transition Advisory Board.

Taggart, E. (2006) *Are You being heard? Strengthening the Voices of Service Users, Patients and Carers in National Health and Social Care Policy Making.* A discussion paper on behalf of the 'National Voices' working group, December. London: 'National Voices' Working Group.

Taggart, E. (2007) *National Voices: A Proposal to Strengthen the Voices of Service Users, Patients and Carers in National Health and Social Care Policy Making.* London: 'National Voices' Working Group.

Taylor, D. and Bury, M. (2007) 'Chronic Illness, Expert Patients and Care Transition'. *Sociology of Health and Illness,* 29 (1): 27–45.

Thompson, S. and Hoggett, P. (2001) 'The Emotional Dynamics of Deliberative Democracy'. *Policy and Politics,* 29 (3): 351–63.

Thornton, S. (2006) 'Democratic Control is Essential'. *British Medical Journal,* 333: 251–2.

Thorlsby, R. and Turner, P. (2007) Choice and Equity: PCT Survey. London: King's Fund.

Townsend, P. and Davidson, N. (1988) 'Introduction'. In *Inequalities in Health: the Black Report*. P. Townsend and N. Davidson (eds). London: Penguin Books.

Tritter, J. and Brittain, I. (2006) 'The NHS Centre for Involvement: Building Excellence in Patient and Public Involvement'. In *Health Democracy: The future of Involvement in Health and Social Care*, E Andersson, J Tritter and R Wilson (eds.) London: Involve, University of Warwick.

Tritter, J.Q., and McCallum, A. (2006) 'The Snakes and Ladders of User Involvement: Moving Beyond Arnstein'. *Health Policy*, 76: 156–68.

Tudor-Hart, J. 'The Inverse Care Law'. *Lancet*, 1971: 405–12.

UK PHA (2007) *Comments on the Stakeholder Consultation on NICE Guidance, Public Health Intervention – Health Inequalities*. Accessed www.ukpha.org.uk 19 March 2007.

University of Surrey (1982) *CHCs in the SW Thames Region*: A survey of members conducted by students on the Dip/Msc in social research, Department of Sociology. Guildford, University of Surrey.

Walsh, P. (2002) *Cock up or Conspiracy? Policy development and change management in the NHS: the case of community health councils*. Dissertation for MBA in Health Services Management, University of Hull.

Wanless, D. (2002) *Securing Our Future Health: Taking a Long-term View*. Final Report. London: Stationery Office.

Warburton, D. (2006) *Evaluation of Your Health, Your Care, Your Say: An Independent Report Commissioned by the Department of Health*. London: Department of Health.

Watts, G. (2003) 'Second coming for patient power', *British Medical Journal*, 326: 520, 8 March 2003.

Webster, C. (1996) *The Health Service since the war. Volume II. Government and the British National Health Service 1958–1979*. London: Stationery Office.

Webster, C. (2002) *The NHS: A Political History*. Oxford: Oxford University Press.

Welsh Assembly Government (2006) *Copying Letters to Patients Initiative – Results of Pilot Projects and Next Steps*. WHC (2006) 042. Cardiff Welsh Assembly Government.

Welsh Office (1989) *Welsh Health Planning Forum: Strategic Intent and Direction for the NHS in Wales*. Cardiff: Welsh Office.

Which? (2005) *Which Choice? Health: Policy Paper*. London: Which?

WHO (2006) *Ninth Futures Forum on Health Systems Governance and Public Participation*. Amsterdam, the Netherlands, 10–11 October 2005. Copenhagen: World Health Organization Europe.

Wilkinson, R.G. (2005) *The Impact of Inequality – How to Make Sick Societies Healthier*. Abingdon: Routledge.

Wilmot, S. (2004) 'Foundation Trusts and the Problem of Legitimacy'. *Healthcare Analysis*, 12 (2) 157–69.

Winkler, F. (1989) *Community/consumer Representation in the NHS with Specific Reference to CHCs – Discussion Paper*. London: the Greater London Association of Community Health Councils.

Index